Introductory Guide to
Cardiac Catheterization

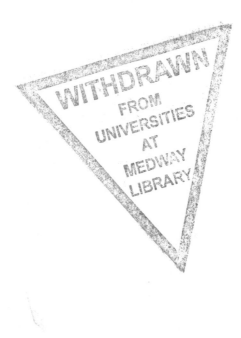

Introductory Guide to Cardiac Catheterization

Editors

Ronnier J. Aviles, M.D.
Cardiovascular Branch
National Heart, Lung, and Blood
 Institute
National Institutes of Health
Bethesda, Maryland

Adrian W. Messerli, M.D.
Department of Interventional
 Cardiology
Washington University School of
 Medicine
St. Louis, Missouri

Arman T. Askari, M.D.
Division of Cardiology
University Hospitals of Cleveland
Case Western Reserve University
Cleveland, Ohio

Marc S. Penn, M.D., Ph.D.
Department of Cardiovascular
 Medicine
The Cleveland Clinic Foundation
Cleveland, Ohio

Eric J. Topol, M.D.
Department of Cardiovascular
 Medicine
The Cleveland Clinic Foundation
Cleveland, Ohio

LIPPINCOTT WILLIAMS & WILKINS
A **Wolters Kluwer** Company
Philadelphia · Baltimore · New York · London
Buenos Aires · Hong Kong · Sydney · Tokyo

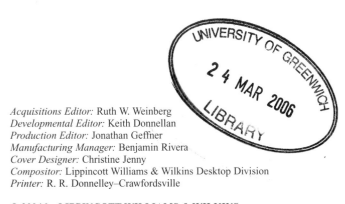

Acquisitions Editor: Ruth W. Weinberg
Developmental Editor: Keith Donnellan
Production Editor: Jonathan Geffner
Manufacturing Manager: Benjamin Rivera
Cover Designer: Christine Jenny
Compositor: Lippincott Williams & Wilkins Desktop Division
Printer: R. R. Donnelley–Crawfordsville

© 2004 by LIPPINCOTT WILLIAMS & WILKINS
530 Walnut Street
Philadelphia, PA 19106 USA
LWW.com

Printed in the USA

Library of Congress Cataloging-in-Publication Data

Introductory guide to cardiac catheterization / [edited by] Ronnier J. Aviles ... [et al.].
    p. ; cm.
    Includes bibliographical references and index.
    ISBN: 0-7817-5202-7
  1. Cardiac catheterization—Handbooks, manuals, etc.
    [DNLM: 1. Heart Catheterization—methods. WG 141.5.C2 I61 2004] I. Aviles, Ronnier J.
RC683.5.C25 I588 2004
616.1¢20754—dc22
                           2003066074

10 9 8 7 6 5 4 3 2 1

To our families for their continuous and faithful support . . . Jennifer, Sandra, Ronnier, Sr., Emily, Mia, Veronica, Jamie, Amanda, Alexa, and Jacob.

CONTENTS

CONTRIBUTING AUTHORS

Sorin J. Brener, M.D.
Department of Medicine, Ohio State University, Columbus, Ohio;
Department of Cardiology, The Cleveland Clinic Foundation,
Cleveland, Ohio

B. Keith Ellis, M.D.
Division of Cardiology, University of Texas Health Sciences Center;
Division of Cardiology, Memorial Hermann Hospital, Houston,
Texas

Hitinder S. Gurm, M.B.B.Ch.
Department of Cardiovascular Medicine, Division of Interventional
Cardiology, The Cleveland Clinic Foundation, Cleveland, Ohio

Frederick A. Heupler, Jr., M.D.
Deartment of Cardiovascular Disease, The Cleveland Clinic
Foundation, Cleveland, Ohio

Robert E. Hobbs, M.D.
Kaufman Center for Heart Failure, The Cleveland Clinic
Foundation, Cleveland, Ohio

David Lee, M.D.
Department of Cardiovascular Medicine, Division of Interventional
Cardiology, The Cleveland Clinic Foundation, Cleveland, Ohio

A. Michael Lincoff, M.D.
Department of Cardiovascular Medicine, Division of Interventional
Cardiology, The Cleveland Clinic Foundation, Cleveland, Ohio

Anjli Maroo, M.D.
Department of Cardiovascular Medicine, The Cleveland Clinic
Foundation, Cleveland, Ohio

J. Christopher Merritt, M.D.
Department of Cardiology, Emory University, Atlanta, Georgia

Niranjan Seshadri, M.D.
Department of Cardiology, Harvard University Medical School;
Beth Israel Deaconess Medical Center, Boston, Massachusetts

Michael R. Tamberella III, M.D.
Department of Cardiology, University of Massachusetts Medical
School, Worcester, Massachusetts

Wilson H. Tang, M.D.
Department of Cardiovascular Medicine, The Cleveland Clinic Foundation, Cleveland, Ohio

Deepak Vivekananthan, M.D.
Department of Cardiovascular Medicine, Division of Interventional Cardiology, The Cleveland Clinic Foundation, Cleveland, Ohio

Michael Yen, M.D.
Department of Cardiovascular Medicine, Division of Interventional Cardiology, The Cleveland Clinic Foundation, Cleveland, Ohio

FOREWORD

Consider you are a novice to the catheterization laboratory. Apparently, you got hold of *Introductory Guide to Cardiac Catheterization*. Now, all you have to do is retire for an afternoon and study it. You will still be a novice, but you will be an enlightened and knowledgeable novice.

The authors, primarily cardiology fellows instrumental for the content and format of the manual, look at the challenging, sometimes frustrating, but mostly gratifying work in the cardiac catheterization laboratory from the front end. I look at it from the back end, with the perspective of a lifelong career, and I see things exactly as they do. This comes as close as anything to guaranteeing that the content of this book is intelligible, valuable, and lasting.

In a succinct style and a condensed format, the authors report from the scene. It is apparent that they have been in the midst of the action for a while; that they have been wide awake while being there; and that they have been blessed with the particular talent to grasp things, weigh them, and convey them. Of course, the sedimented experiences of the senior authors transpire here and there, particularly when pearls are pointed out that give away the old crack. For instance, the importance of the conus branch of the right coronary artery is highlighted. The conus branch is often missed when it takes off separately from the right coronary artery, and it may be the only contributor to an occluded left anterior descending coronary artery. Or it is recommended to keep attempts to pass a stenosed aortic valve in time with systole. In diastole, it is indeed impossible to pass the valve as it is closed; trivial, but blatantly ignored by most of us.

The manual is made for readers or browsers. The readers will prevail, as this is one of those books that is hard to put down. Hence, most will start reading nonchalantly about how to prepare themselves and the patients for what has to be done in the catheterization laboratory. Then they will casually settle down more comfortably to learn all they need to learn, but not a thing more, about radiation protection and the basic material, just before diving into some tricks of the trade explained in plain words and with high-quality photographs and illustrations wherever pertinent. By now, they will be practically oblivious to what is going on around them. Only the lazy ones will skip the somewhat more demanding chapter on hemodynamics, muttering excuses such as "in my place, the computer does this." This chapter has been the kernel of the thick-belly books on cardiac catheterization of yesteryear. It still needs to be there, but it needs to be there in a lean and stripped-down version such as what is found in Chapter 6. One certainly should resist the temptation to skip the final short chapter about the after care, because this usually is more important for the patient than the brief intermezzo in the catheterization laboratory, most of which he or she missed anyhow.

I also recommend this compendium for cardiologists in the phase of only toying with the idea of commencing a career in the catheterization laboratory. They will be reminded that the video game–like thrill in finding the artery and being able to engage the coronary ostium in a reasonable time is but the tip of the iceberg. What lies beneath is tough, partly repetitious, and at times boring routine work with more immediate responsibility than many of us might care to bear. When pioneers like Cournand, Sones, and Judkins introduced diagnostic cardiac catheterization and Rubio-Alvarez, Rashkind, King, and Gruentzig added a therapeutic scent to it, they created a field of action for a new breed of doctor: a mixture between the internist with a big brain and the hands in the pockets and the gung-ho surgeon with big guts and the hands in everything but the pockets. *Introductory Guide to Cardiac Catheterization* will help you to find out whether you are one of that league or whether it is worth (and safe) for you to try to become one. Enjoy it!

Bernhard Meier, M.D.
Professor and Head of Cardiology
Swiss Cardiovascular Center Bern
University Hospital
Bern, Switzerland

PREFACE

For a newcomer, the catheterization laboratory can be an unsettling place. Certain patients may be extremely ill, and routine procedures can suddenly become protracted and complicated. Because the margin of error is thin and the atmosphere is frequently tense, students may quickly be overwhelmed and frustrated. The primary authors and editors of this manual are cardiology fellows who remember well what it was like to enter the cath lab for the first time. With this experience still fresh in our minds, our goal was to provide a comprehensive, yet practical guide for physicians, physicians-in-training, and cath lab nurses and personnel embarking on a career in coronary angiography. *Introductory Guide to Cardiac Catheterization* was specifically designed with an easy-to-read format that includes highlighted "pearls," American College of Cardiology/American Heart Association (ACC/AHA) guidelines, two-color illustrations (including carefully constructed schematics of standard coronary projections), and special "troubleshooting" sections that provide potential solutions for frequently encountered problems. We intended this manual to fit easily into a lab coat, so that it can be taken on patient rounds or into the lab and serve as a quick reference in the middle of an otherwise hectic day.

We gratefully acknowledge the contributions of our teachers at The Cleveland Clinic, who went above and beyond in their tutelage and mentoring, and who have supported and encouraged us as we developed this manual. Any deficiencies herein are solely ours! We also acknowledge Marion Tomasko, Suzanne Turner, Charlene Surace, and Mary Ann Citraro, who patiently put up with us as they worked tirelessly on the graphics. Finally, a special nod of thanks to each of the cardiology fellows in the graduating class of 2003 who contributed.

On behalf of the contributors, we genuinely hope that you find this to be a useful guide as you learn and gain proficiency in this challenging yet rewarding (and fun) field.

We appreciate your feedback. If you have any suggestions for improvements or any corrections, please address your comments to: cathmanual@hotmail.com.

Ronnier J. Aviles, M.D.
Adrian W. Messerli, M.D.
Arman T. Askari, M.D.

1. PRE-CATH

Anjli Maroo and Sorin J. Brener

Basic Evaluation
Indications for Cardiac Catheterization
Complications of Coronary Angiography
Medication Considerations Prior to Coronary Angiography

The use of cardiac catheterization for both diagnostic and therapeutic purposes continues to grow, approaching 2 million procedures
performed annually in the United States. Due to the inherent risks
associated with this invasive procedure, operators who perform
angiograms must be intimately familiar with the indications, contraindications, and potential complications associated with
catheterization. Thorough preprocedural evaluation facilitates the
appropriate selection of candidates for catheterization and the identification of patients at highest risk for complications.

BASIC EVALUATION

Careful inquiry into the presenting symptoms and signs is an essential component of the precatheterization evaluation. In addition to
establishing the indication for catheterization, the clinical presentation guides the selection of techniques employed during catheterization, including coronary angiography, hemodynamic measurements,
left ventriculography, aortography, right heart catheterization, provocative pharmacologic challenge, intraaortic balloon pump placement, biopsy, and percutaneous coronary intervention.

Concomitant medical conditions should be determined and
addressed prior to catheterization (Table 1-1). Severe thrombocytopenia or coagulopathy may render the patient ineligible for
catheterization. In those with a prior history of heparin-induced
thrombocytopenia, heparin-free solutions and flushes should be prepared. Alternate forms of anticoagulation, such as direct thrombin
inhibitors, may be preferable for percutaneous intervention. In
patients with chronic renal insufficiency, renal function should be
optimized prior to catheterization.

Patients with severe lower-extremity arterial disease may require
catheterization via the brachial or radial artery. A history of abdominal or thoracic aortic aneurysm or prior aortic dissection may also
favor brachial or radial artery access. A history of claudication in

TABLE 1-1. PREPROCEDURAL CONSIDERATIONS

Bleeding disorders
Prior stroke
Comorbid medical conditions
   Chronic renal insufficiency
   Diabetes mellitus
   Peripheral vascular disease
   Hypertension
   Anemia
   Thrombocytopenia
   Cancer
   Pulmonary disease
   Liver disease
Known contrast allergy
Heparin-induced thrombocytopenia
Prior cardiac catheterizations and/or surgeries
Results of echocardiogram, stress test, and electrocardiogram

one lower extremity should be taken into account when selecting the arterial access site.

In patients with known preexisting coronary disease, **detailed knowledge of all prior catheterizations, percutaneous interventions, and cardiac surgeries is imperative**. If possible, films of prior catheterizations should be reviewed for comparison. Knowledge of prior peripheral vascular interventions and surgeries is also required to plan arterial access.

Medication allergies should be documented prior to the procedure. Patients with a history of contrast media allergy in particular require special consideration. Latex allergy is not a contraindication to cardiac catheterization. The catheterization laboratory should be notified of the allergy and should be prepared to receive the patient as the first case of the day. Special latex-free equipment should be utilized.

A focused physical exam is a prerequisite of catheterizations. Signs of congestive heart failure, such as rales, jugular venous distension, an S_3, significant murmurs, or peripheral edema should be noted. A careful examination of peripheral pulses and search for arterial bruits will influence the choice of arterial access site and serve as a helpful comparison when assessing for postprocedural vascular complications.

Standard laboratory evaluation includes assessing **electrolytes, blood urea nitrogen, serum creatinine, blood glucose, complete blood count, partial thromboplastin time and prothrombin time**. These laboratory tests should be current (i.e., within 1 month of the procedure). Similarly, a current **electrocardiogram** should be assessed. Evidence of ischemia, prior myocardial infarction (MI), rhythm disturbances, and chamber enlargement/hypertrophy should be noted. If a prior **echocardiogram** is available, preprocedural knowledge of left ventricular systolic or diastolic dysfunction, significant valvular disease, and aortic abnormalities is often helpful. Similarly, if the results of a prior **stress test** is available, the operator should become familiar with areas of ischemia and scar.

INDICATIONS FOR CARDIAC CATHETERIZATION

The decision to proceed with diagnostic cardiac catheterization is based on a careful assessment of the risk–benefit ratio for the procedure. The most current guidelines for diagnostic coronary angiography, reported by a joint task force of the American College of Cardiology and the American Heart Association (ACC/AHA), divide the indications for coronary angiography into three classes (Table 1-2). Class I indications are conditions for which there is evidence and/or general agreement that the procedure is useful and effective. Class II indications are conditions for which there is conflicting evidence and/or a divergence of opinion about the usefulness/efficacy of performing the procedure. Class III indications are conditions for which there is evidence and/or general agreement that the procedure is not useful/effective and, in some cases, may be harmful.

The role of diagnostic catheterization during acute MI has grown dramatically in the past decade. In the 1991 ACC/AHA guidelines, there were no class I indications for coronary angiography during the acute phases of an MI. Now coronary angiography is used frequently to evaluate patients presenting with acute MI for potential percutaneous or surgical revascularization. The 1999 ACC/AHA guidelines stratify the use of coronary angiography during acute MI by the type of MI [ST elevation or new left bundle branch block (LBBB) versus non-ST elevation] and by phase of treatment (early versus in-hospital versus risk-stratification stage). **Emergent coronary angiography with the intent to perform primary percutaneous coronary intervention is most applicable to patients presenting within 12 hours of an acute ST elevation or new LBBB MI. This strategy can also be applied to patients with (a) non–ST-elevation MI who have persistent or recurrent symptoms despite optimal medical therapy or (b) patients younger than 75 years with ST elevation, new LBBB, or non–ST-elevation MI complicated by cardiogenic shock or hemodynamic instability.** During the in-hospital phase following all types of MI, recurrent ischemia, mechanical complications, and hemodynamic instability all warrant coronary angiography. Coronary angiography should be considered in patients with post-MI LV systolic dysfunction, clinical heart failure, and malignant arrhythmias. Coronary angiography

TABLE 1-2. INDICATIONS FOR CORONARY ANGIOGRAPHY

Class I

Unstable Coronary Syndromes
    Unstable angina/ACS refractory to medical therapy, or recurrent symptoms after initial medical therapy
    Unstable angina/ACS at high- or intermediate-risk for adverse outcome
    Unstable angina/ACS initially at low-level, short-term risk, with subsequent high-risk noninvasive testing
    Prinzmetal angina
    Suspected for abrupt or subacute stent thrombosis after PCI

Angina
    High-risk features on noninvasive testing
    CCS class III or IV angina on medical therapy
    Recurrent angina 9 months after PCI

Acute Myocardial Infarction
    Intended PCI in acute ST-elevation or new BBB MI
        Within 12 h of symptom onset
        Ischemic symptoms persisting after 12 h of symptom onset
        Cardiogenic shock within 36 h of symptom onset
    Angiography in non–ST-elevation MI
        Persistent or recurrent symptomatic ischemia with or without associated ECG changes
        Associated shock, severe pulmonary congestion, persistent hypotension
        Resting ischemia or ischemia provoked by minimal exertion following infarction
        Before repair of a mechanical complication of MI
    Risk-stratification phase (for all types of MI)
        Abnormal low-level noninvasive stress test

Perioperative Risk Stratification for Noncardiac Surgery
    High-risk features on noninvasive testing
    Unstable angina
    Equivocal noninvasive test result in patient with high-risk features undergoing high-risk surgery

Congestive Heart Failure
    Systolic dysfunction associated with angina, regional wall motion abnormalities, or ischemia on noninvasive testing
    Prior to cardiac transplantation
    Mechanical complications of MI

Other Conditions
    Valve surgery in patients with angina, multiple-risk factors for CAD, or high-risk features on noninvasive testing
    Correction of congenital heart disease in patients with angina, high-risk features on noninvasive testing, or coronary anomalies
    After successful resuscitation from sudden cardiac death, sustained monomorphic ventricular tachycardia, or unsustained polymorphic ventricular tachycardia
    Infective endocarditis with evidence of coronary embolization
    Diseases of the aorta necessitating knowledge of concomitant coronary disease
    Hypertrophic cardiomyopathy with angina

(continued)

TABLE 1-2. *(continued)*

Class II

Angina
  CCS class III or IV that improves to class I or II on medical therapy
  CCS class I or II that fails to improve with medical therapy
  Progressive abnormality on noninvasive testing
  Patient who cannot be risk stratified by other means
  Recurrent angina within 12 mo of CABG
  Recurrent angina poorly controlled with medical therapy after revascularization

Acute Myocardial Infarction
  Suspected to have occurred by a mechanism other than thrombotic occlusion
    of atherosclerotic plaque
  Coronary embolism, arteritis, trauma, coronary spasm
  Failed thrombolysis with planned rescue PCI
  Post MI with LVEF <40%, CHF, prior revascularization, or malignant
    arrhythmias
  CHF during acute episode with subsequent demonstration of LVEF >40%
  Risk-stratification phase
    CHF during hospitalization
    Inability to perform exercise stress test, with LVEF <45%

Perioperative Risk Stratification for Noncardiac Surgery
  Planned vascular surgery with multiple intermediate-risk factors
  Abnormal stress test without high-risk factors
  Equivocal noninvasive testing in patient with intermediate-risk factors
    undergoing high-risk surgery
  Urgent noncardiac surgery while recovering from an acute MI
  Perioperative MI

Other Conditions
  Systolic LV dysfunction with unexplained cause after noninvasive testing
  Episodic CHF with normal systolic LV function, with suspicion for ischemia-
    mediated LV dysfunction
  Recent blunt chest trauma and suspicion for acute MI
  Before surgery for aortic dissection/aneurysm in a patient without known CAD
  Periodic follow-up after cardiac transplantation
  Perioperative MI
  Asymptomatic patients with Kawasaki disease and coronary artery aneurysms
    on echocardiography

ACS, acute coronary syndrome; BBB, bundle branch block; CABG, coronary artery bypass graft; CAD, coronary artery disease; CCS, Canadian Cardiovascular Society (classification); CHF, congestive heart failure; ECG, electrocardiogram; LV, left ventricular; LVEF, LV ejection fraction; MI, myocardial infarction; PCI, percutaneous coronary intervention.

Adapted from Scanlon PJ, Faxon DP, Audet AM, et al. ACC/AHA guidelines for coronary angiography: Executive summary and recommendations. A report of the American College of Cardiology/American Heart Association Task Force on Practice Guidelines (Committee on Coronary Angiography) developed in collaboration with the Society for Cardiac Angiography and Interventions. *Circulation* 1999;99:2345–2357.

is indicated during the risk-stratification phase following all types of MI in patients with ischemia provoked by stress testing, moderate or severe left ventricular systolic dysfunction, or inability to perform stress testing.

In patients with known or suspected coronary disease who are experiencing typical angina, the Canadian Cardiovascular Society classification of angina is a useful tool for gauging the severity of symptoms (Table 1-3). Patients with severe symptoms (CCS class III or IV), despite optimal medical therapy, should undergo coronary angiography. Presence of high-risk criteria on noninvasive testing (Table 1-4) should also prompt coronary angiography in patients with known or suspected coronary disease, regardless of symptom severity. Patients with deterioration on serial noninvasive testing or patients with accelerating (crescendo) angina despite medical therapy should also be considered for angiography, even if noninvasive testing does not demonstrate high-risk factors. It is important to use objective measures such as noninvasive testing to risk-stratify patients with stable angina and who respond well to medical therapy. **Routine angiography in asymptomatic patients without evidence of ischemia is not advised**. Patients who are successfully resuscitated from sudden cardiac death (without a readily identifiable cause) have a high probability of underlying coronary disease and should undergo cardiac catheterization.

Atypical or nonspecific chest pain is infrequently due to myocardial ischemia. There are, however, several rare causes of ischemia that should be entertained in the differential diagnosis of atypical chest pain. These include Prinzmetal angina, cocaine abuse, syndrome X, pericarditis, myocarditis, coronary embolus, and aortic dissection. Noncardiac causes of chest pain include costochondritis, pleuritis, pulmonary embolus, and esophageal disorders. Due to the broad spectrum of possible etiologies for atypical chest pain, coronary angiography should be reserved for patients who demonstrate high-risk findings on noninvasive testing.

TABLE 1-3. **CANADIAN CARDIOVASCULAR SOCIETY CLASSIFICATION OF ANGINA**

Classification	Definition
I	Ordinary physical activity does not cause angina
II	Slight limitation of ordinary activity (walking more than two blocks or climbing more than one flight of stairs)
III	Marked limitation of ordinary physical activity (walking one to two blocks or climbing one flight of stairs)
IV	Inability to carry on any activity without discomfort

TABLE 1-4. NONINVASIVE TEST RESULTS PREDICTING HIGH RISK FOR ADVERSE OUTCOME

Severe left ventricular dysfunction
High-risk Duke treadmill score (≤ -11)
Severe exercise-induced left ventricular dysfunction
Large stress-induced perfusion defect (particularly if anterior)
Stress-induced, moderately-sized multiple perfusion defects
Large, fixed perfusion defect with left ventricular dilation or increased lung uptake
Stress-induced, moderately-sized perfusion defect with left ventricular dilation or increased lung uptake
Echocardiographic wall motion abnormality (involving more than two segments) developing at a low dose of dobutamine or at a low heart rate
Stress echocardiographic evidence of extensive ischemia

LVEF, left ventricular ejection fraction.
Adapted from Scanlon PJ, Faxon DP, Audet AM, et al. ACC/AHA guidelines for coronary angiography: Executive summary and recommendations. A report of the American College of Cardiology/American Heart Association Task Force on Practice Guidelines (Committee on Coronary Angiography) developed in collaboration with the Society for Cardiac Angiography and Interventions. *Circulation* 1999;99:2345–2537.

Patients presenting with unstable angina can be divided into high-risk, intermediate-risk, and low-risk categories (Table 1-5). High- or intermediate-risk factors in patients refractory to adequate medical therapy or with recurrent symptoms after initial stabilization may prompt emergent catheterization. Patients with low-risk factors may be further risk-stratified with noninvasive testing prior to consideration of catheterization.

Development of ischemia after percutaneous coronary intervention may occur via acute or subacute stent thrombosis (less than 48 hours) or via in-stent restenosis (3 to 6 months). Surgical revascularization may be complicated by graft obstruction in the immediate perioperative period or by graft disease that develops over time. **Suspected stent thrombosis warrants consideration of immediate catheterization and possible percutaneous coronary intervention**. Patients with recurrent angina or high-risk factors on noninvasive testing within 9 months of successful percutaneous intervention or 12 months following coronary artery bypass graft surgery are also suitable candidates for coronary angiography.

In patients who are undergoing surgery for valvular disease and are at increased risk for concomitant coronary disease, coronary angiography is recommended. Presence of chest pain, ischemia on noninvasive testing, or multiple risk factors for coronary disease all constitute class I indications for catheterization. Patients who have infective endocarditis and demonstrate evidence of coronary embolism also should undergo coronary angiography. In patients with aortic valve endocarditis, particular care must be paid during catheter

TABLE 1-5. SHORT-TERM RISKS FOR DEATH OR MYOCARDIAL INFARCTION IN PATIENTS WITH UNSTABLE ANGINA

High Risk
    Prolonged (>20 min) pain at rest, ongoing
    Pulmonary edema
    Dynamic ST changes (>1 mm) or positive cardiac troponins
    New or worsening mitral regurgitation
    Third heart sound
    Hypotension

Intermediate Risk
    Prolonged (>20 min) pain at rest, now resolved
    Angina at rest (>20 min) or relieved by rest, or with nitroglycerin
    Nocturnal angina
    Dynamic T-wave changes
    New-onset CCS class III or IV angina within the past 2 wk, with moderate to
       high likelihood of CAD
    Pathologic Q waves or ST depression (<1 mm) in multiple leads
    Age >65 yr

Low Risk
    Increased frequency, severity, or duration of angina
    Angina provoked at lower threshold
    New-onset angina 2 wk to 2 mo before presentation
    Normal or unchanged ECG

CAD, coronary artery disease; CCS, Canadian Cardiovascular Society (classification); ECG, electrocardiogram.
Adapted from Scanlon PJ, Faxon DP, Audet AM, et al. ACC/AHA guidelines for coronary angiography: Executive summary and recommendations. A report of the American College of Cardiology/American Heart Association Task Force on Practice Guidelines (Committee on Coronary Angiography) developed in collaboration with the Society for Cardiac Angiography and Interventions. *Circulation* 1999;99:2345–2537.

manipulation to avoid disrupting the vegetation, which could result in an embolic episode.

The presence of left ventricular systolic dysfunction is a poor prognostic sign. Any patient with congestive heart failure, reversible ischemia on noninvasive testing, or regional wall motion abnormalities should be evaluated for coronary disease by angiography. Systolic dysfunction that is unexplained by noninvasive testing should be further investigated by angiography.

It is equally important to be aware of conditions for which angiography is not recommended (Table 1-6). Patients who refuse or who are ineligible for revascularization should not undergo coronary angiography in the setting of nonspecific chest pain, stable angina, unstable angina, or MI. Similarly, if revascularization is unlikely to improve symptom control or longevity, coronary angiography should not be performed.

The only absolute contraindication to coronary angiography is the patient's refusal to undergo the procedure. There are, however, several relative contraindications (Table 1-7). A his-

TABLE 1-6. CLASS III INDICATIONS FOR CORONARY ANGIOGRAPHY

Unstable Angina
  Symptoms suggestive of unstable angina but without objective signs of ische-
    mia and with a normal coronary angiogram within the past 5 yr
  Unstable angina in a patient who is not a revascularization candidate or in
    whom revascularization will not improve the quality or duration of life
  Unstable angina in a postbypass patient who is not a revascularization
    candidate

Angina and Coronary Artery Disease
  Angina in a patient who refuses revascularization
  Screening test for CAD in asymptomatic patients
  Coronary calcification detected on fluoroscopy or electron beam computed
    tomography
  Nonspecific chest pain with normal noninvasive testing
  Routine angiography in an asymptomatic patient after PCI or CABG

Myocardial Infarction: ST-segment Elevation or New LBBB
  Patient is beyond 12-h symptom onset with no evidence of ongoing ischemia
  Postthrombolytic therapy with no evidence of ongoing ischemia
  Routine angiography and PTCA within 24 h of thrombolytic therapy

All Myocardial Infarction: Hospital Management and Risk-Stratification Phase
  Patient is not a revascularization candidate or refuses revascularization

Perioperative Risk Stratification for Noncardiac Surgery
  Low-risk surgery with known CAD and no high-risk factors on noninvasive
    testing
  Asymptomatic after revascularization with excellent exercise capacity (>7
    METS)
  Mild stable angina, good left ventricular function, with no high-risk factors on
    noninvasive testing
  Part of work-up for renal, liver, or lung transplant, with no high-risk factors on
    noninvasive testing

Valvular Heart Disease
  Prior to surgery for infective endocarditis in a patient lacking risk factors for
    CAD or evidence of coronary embolization
  Routine angiography in a patient not being assessed for surgery

BBB, bundle branch block; CABG, coronary artery bypass graft; CAD, coronary artery
disease; LBBB, left bundle branch block; METS, metabolic equivalent; PCI,
percutaneous coronary intervention; PTCA, percutaneous transluminal coronary
angioplasty.
Adapted from Scanlon PJ, Faxon DP, Audet AM, et al. ACC/AHA guidelines for
coronary angiography: Executive summary and recommendations. A report of the
American College of Cardiology/American Heart Association Task Force on Practice
Guidelines (Committee on Coronary Angiography) developed in collaboration with the
Society for Cardiac Angiography and Interventions. *Circulation* 1999;99:2345–2357.

tory of acute or chronic renal failure prior to catheterization is a
concern. Contrast-induced or atheroembolic renal failure incurred
during catheterization may significantly worsen preexisting renal
dysfunction. Gastrointestinal bleeding or unexplained anemia is a
noteworthy concern, especially if high-dose anticoagulation will be

TABLE 1-7. **RELATIVE CONTRAINDICATIONS TO CORONARY ANGIOGRAPHY**

Acute renal failure
Chronic renal failure due to diabetes mellitus
Active gastrointestinal bleeding
Unexplained fever
Untreated active infection
Acute stroke
Severe anemia
Severe uncontrolled hypertension
Severe symptomatic electrolyte imbalance
Refusal to cooperate or accept revascularization or surgery
Concomitant severe illness reducing life expectancy
Digitalis intoxication
Anaphylactoid reaction to angiographic contrast media
Decompensated heart failure or acute pulmonary edema
Severe coagulopathy
Aortic valve endocarditis

Adapted from Scanlon PJ, Faxon DP, Audet AM, et al. ACC/AHA guidelines for coronary angiography. A report of the American College of Cardiology/American Heart Association Task Force on practice guidelines (Committee on Coronary Angiography). Developed in collaboration with the Society for Cardiac Angiography and Interventions. *J Am Cardiol* 1999;33:1756–1824.

required for potential percutaneous coronary intervention following diagnostic angiography. Uncontrolled hypertension increases the risk of complications related to the arterial puncture site. Patients with decompensated heart failure may not be able to tolerate lying flat and may suffer further decompensation from the contrast load.

COMPLICATIONS OF CORONARY ANGIOGRAPHY

The risk of major complications following diagnostic angiography is generally less than 2%. However, several comorbid conditions significantly increase this baseline risk (Table 1-8). Assessment of the patient's risk for complications is an important determinant of whether the procedure can be performed on an outpatient basis. Several factors favor short-term hospitalization after catheterization, including hydration for patients with chronic renal insufficiency (Table 1-9).

Obtaining informed consent for the catheterization is an integral part of preparing the patient. This discussion should include a thorough explanation of the indication for the procedure, the risks of administering conscious sedation, the risks and benefits of the catheterization procedure, and the potential need for emergency coronary artery bypass graft surgery. Although the risk of an adverse event for an individual patient does depend on the patient's comorbidities, the operator's experience, the type of procedure, and

TABLE 1-8. PREDICTORS OF MAJOR COMPLICATIONS[a]

Predictor	Odds Ratio (95% Confidence Interval)
Moribund[b]	10.22 (3.77, 27.76)
Shock	6.52 (4.18, 10.18)
Acute myocardial infarction (onset <24 h)	4.03 (2.61, 6.21)
Renal insufficiency	3.30 (2.39, 4.55)
Cardiomyopathy	3.29 (2.23, 4.86)
Aortic valve disease	2.72 (2.02, 3.66)
Mitral valve disease	2.33 (1.76, 3.08)
Congestive heart failure	2.22 (1.71, 2.90)
New York Heart Association functional class	10.22 (3.77, 27.76)
Class I	1.0
Class II	1.15 (0.94, 1.41)
Class III	1.32 (0.92, 1.51)
Class IV	1.52 (1.16, 1.74)
Hypertension	1.45 (1.22, 1.73)
Unstable angina	1.42 (1.16, 1.74)
Outpatient/inpatient	0.63 (0.52, 0.76)

[a]Based on 58,332 procedures.
[b]Moribund indicates a patient who responds poorly to therapy due to a life-threatening condition, myocardial infarction, major complication, or any adverse event listed in Table 1-7.
Adapted from Scanlon PJ, Faxon DP, Audet AM, et al. ACC/AHA guidelines for coronary angiography. A report of the American College of Cardiology/American Heart Association Task Force on practice guidelines (Committee on Coronary Angiography). Developed in collaboration with the Society for Cardiac Angiography and Interventions. *J Am Cardiol* 1999;33:1756–1824.

TABLE 1-9. FACTORS FAVORING HOSPITALIZATION FOLLOWING CARDIAC CATHETERIZATION

High risk for vascular complications
Mechanical prosthetic valve
Left ventricular ejection fraction <35%
Anticoagulation or bleeding diathesis
Uncontrolled hypertension
Brittle diabetes mellitus
Chronic steroid use
History of allergy to contrast media
Severe chronic obstructive pulmonary disease
Age <21 yr or has complex congenital disease
Recent (<1 mo) cerebrovascular accident
Severe ischemia during noninvasive testing
Moderate to severe pulmonary hypertension
Arterial oxygen desaturation

Adapted from Pepine CJ. Coronary angiography and cardiac catheterization. In: Topol EJ, ed. *Textbook of cardiovascular medicine.* Philadelphia: Lippincott Williams & Wilkins, 1998:1935–1956.

the clinical setting in which the procedure is being performed, pooled frequencies of major complications may be used during an informed consent discussion (Table 1-10).

The rate of death complicating coronary angiography has steadily fallen over the past 15 years and is now approximately 0.1%. High-risk factors for periprocedural mortality include advanced age (60 years or older), New York Heart Association functional class IV, severe left main coronary artery disease, and left ventricular systolic dysfunction (ejection fraction less than or equal to 30%). Baseline renal insufficiency with worsening of renal function following catheterization is associated with a particularly high mortality.

Periprocedural MI is fairly uncommon (less than or equal to 0.1%). For those at high risk (e.g., left main coronary artery disease, recent acute coronary syndrome, insulin-dependent diabetes mellitus), cardiac enzymes may be followed after the procedure. **Periprocedural stroke is also uncommon (less than or equal to 0.07%).** Strokes are more common in patients with severe aortic atherosclerosis. In such patients, catheter exchanges may be performed over a guide wire to minimize aortic atheromatous plaque disruption. Patients who undergo catheterization following administration of thrombolytics or who receive high-dose anticoagulation are at increased risk for hemorrhagic stroke.

Local vascular complications, the most frequent complications following catheterization, are discussed in greater detail in Chapters 8 and 9.

The most common allergic reactions encountered during catheterization result from administration of local anesthetic, contrast dye,

TABLE 1-10. RISK OF CARDIAC CATHETERIZATION[a]

Complication	Frequency (%)
Mortality	0.11
Myocardial infarction	0.05
Cerebrovascular accident	0.07
Arrhythmia	0.38
Vascular complications	0.43
Contrast reaction	0.37
Hemodynamic complications	0.26
Perforation of the heart chamber	0.03
Other complications	0.28
Total no. of major complications	1.7

[a]N = 59,792.
Adapted from Noto TJ Jr, et al. Cardiac catheterization 1990: A report of the registry of the Society for Cardiac Angiography and Interventions (SCA&I). *Cathet Cardiovasc Diagn* 1991;24:75–83.

or protamine sulfate. Contrast dye allergies are relatively common. Patients with known dye allergies should be premedicated with corticosteroids and antihistamines, and should receive noniodinated contrast (See Chapter 2.)

Renal dysfunction can result from administration of contrast agents and/or from renal atheroembolic disease. Renal atheroembolic disease complicates approximately 0.15% of cardiac catheterizations. Renal failure due to atheroemboli usually has a prolonged course. Clinical indicators of atheroembolic disease include purple toes, livedo reticularis, systemic or urinary eosinophilia, malaise, anorexia, abdominal pain, and lower extremity pain. Contrast-induced nephropathy and its prevention are discussed in greater detail in Chapter 2.

TROUBLESHOOTING

Patients with renal dysfunction: Patients with any degree of renal impairment need to be well hydrated prior to cardiac catheterization. Hydration with either normal saline or 0.45% saline for 6 to 12 hours before and 12 to 24 hours after the procedure is reasonable. Use of acetylcysteine (Mucomyst 600 mg p.o. b.i.d. starting the day prior to the procedure) in high-risk patients (serum creatinine greater than 2.0 mg/dL) should also be considered. It is important to make patients with renal dysfunction who may require a coronary intervention aware of the possibility of a staged procedure in case this becomes necessary to minimize the contrast load.

In the event of an ischemic complication during the procedure, it is advantageous to have cardiac surgical backup available. The patient and his or her family should be aware of the potential need for coronary artery bypass surgery or percutaneous coronary intervention.

MEDICATION CONSIDERATIONS PRIOR TO CORONARY ANGIOGRAPHY

In patients who are candidates for percutaneous coronary intervention after diagnostic angiography, aspirin 325 mg should be administered on the day of the procedure (Table 1-11). The use of clopidogrel (300 mg loading dose) prior to catheterization may be indicated in patients likely to undergo percutaneous coronary intervention.

TABLE 1-11. PREPROCEDURAL MEDICATION CONSIDERATIONS

Medication	Adjustment
Aspirin	325 mg prior to the procedure
Clopidogrel (Plavix)	300 mg loading dose if there is a high probability of PCI
GPIIb–IIIa inhibitor	Continue if already started; may be started on arrival to lab if PCI planned
Unfractionated heparin	Per discretion of operator
Low-molecular-weight heparin	Per discretion of operator
Warfarin (Coumadin)	Hold for 2–3 days prior to procedure until INR <1.8; heparin or low-molecular-weight heparin can be used if continued anticoagulation is essential
Insulin and hypoglycemics	Hold the morning of the procedure
Metformin (Glucophage)	Hold on the day prior to procedure and resume 2 days after procedure if renal function remains unchanged
Acetylcysteine (Mucomyst)	600 mg p.o. b.i.d. starting the day prior to the procedure for patients with chronic renal dysfunction

INR, international normalized ratio; PCI, percutaneous coronary intervention.

This must be weighed against the possibility that they will require coronary artery bypass graft surgery, which often must be postponed for several days after administration of clopidogrel. **Warfarin should be stopped several days before the procedure. Ideally, the international normalized ratio should be less than 1.8 prior to catheterization.** Heparin (3,000 to 5,000 units i.v.) should be considered for patients undergoing cardiac catheterization via the arm.

Metformin (Glucophage) is eliminated primarily through the kidneys and therefore accumulates in patients with renal insufficiency (glomerular filtration rate of less than 70 mL/min, or serum creatinine greater than 1.6 mg/dL). Contrast media can impair renal function and lead to further retention of metformin, which is known to precipitate the onset of lactic acidosis. The incidence of lactic acidosis associated with metformin, regardless of exposure to contrast media, is 0.03 cases per 1,000 patients per year, and 50% result in death. There is no conclusive evidence to indicate that contrast media precipitates the development of metformin-induced lactic acidosis among patients with normal serum creatinine (less than 1.5 mg/dL). This complication is almost exclusively observed among non–insulin-dependent diabetic patients with abnormal renal function before injection of contrast media. **Metformin should be withheld the day prior to the procedure and restarted 2 days after the procedure if renal function remains unchanged.**

GENERAL SUGGESTED READINGS

Baim DS, Grossman W, eds. *Grossman's cardiac catheterization, angiography, and intervention.* 6th ed. Philadelphia: Lippincott Williams & Wilkins, 2000.

Braunwald E, Zipes DP, Libby P. *Heart disease: a textbook of cardiovascular medicine.* 6th ed. Philadelphia: WB Saunders, 2001.

Pepine CJ, Hill JA, Lambert CR, eds. *Diagnostic and therapeutic cardiac catheterization, 3rd ed.* Baltimore: Williams & Wilkins, 1998.

Peterson KL, Nicod P, eds. *Cardiac catheterization: methods, diagnosis, and therapy.* Philadelphia: WB Saunders, 1997.

Topol EJ, ed. *Textbook of interventional cardiology.* 4th ed. WB Saunders, 2003.

Uretsky BF, ed. *Cardiac catheterization: concepts, techniques and applications.* Malden: Blackwell Science, 1997.

CHAPTER 1 SUGGESTED READINGS

Carrozza JP, Baim DS. *Complications of diagnostic cardiac catheterization.* UpToDate 2002; Version 10.2.

Davidson CJ, Bonow RO. Cardiac catheterization. In: Braunwald E, Zipes DP, Libby P, eds. *Heart disease. A textbook of cardiovascular medicine,* 6th ed. Philadelphia: WB Saunders, 2001:359–386.

La Perna L, Olin JW, Groines D, et al. Ultrasound-guided thrombin injection for the treatment of postcatheterization pseudoaneurysms. *Circulation* 2000;102:2391–2395.

Laskey W, Boyle J, Johnson LW. Multivariable model for prediction of risk of significant complication during diagnostic cardiac catheterization: the Registry Committee of the Society for Cardiac Angiography and Interventions. *Cathet Cardiovasc Diagn* 1993;30:185–190.

Noto TJ, Johnson LW, Krone R, et al. Cardiac catheterization 1990: A report of the registry of the Society for Cardiac Angiography and Interventions. *Cathet Cardiovasc Diagn* 1991;24:75–83.

Ryan TJ, Anderson JL, Antman EM, et al. ACC/AHA guidelines for the management of patients with acute myocardial infarction: a report of the American College of Cardiology/American Heart Association Task Force on Practice Guidelines (Committee on the management of acute myocardial infarction). *J Am Coll Cardiol* 1996;28:1328–1428.

Scanlon PJ, Faxon DP, Audet AM, et al. ACC/AHA guidelines for coronary angiography: executive summary and recommendations. A report of the American College of Cardiology/American Heart Association Task Force on Practice Guidelines (Committee on Coronary Angiography) developed in collaboration with the Society for Cardiac Angiography and Interventions. *Circulation* 1999;99:2345–2357.

Wong T, Detsky AS. Preoperative risk assessment for patients having peripheral vascular surgery. *Ann Intern Med* 1992;116:743–753.

2. SETTING UP THE LAB

Michael Yen and Sorin J. Brener

Prior to the patient's arrival to the catheterization laboratory, the catheterization team should verify that all monitoring, recording, and resuscitation equipment are properly functioning. Continuous monitoring of the patient's electrocardiogram (ECG) upon the patient's arrival to the catheterization laboratory is indispensable since it can quickly identify any arrhythmias, conduction abnormalities, or evidence of ischemia. An automated blood pressure cuff and continuous pulse oximetry are also necessary. Resuscitation equipment such as intubation trays and defibrillators should be tested and placed nearby. If a patient is unable to urinate lying flat or if a long cardiac catheterization is expected, a urinary catheter should be placed.

PREPROCEDURAL SEDATION

In nonemergent situations, a detailed discussion with the patient and family explaining the cardiac catheterization procedure, potential complications, and alternative diagnostic options will help to alleviate any anxiety prior to the procedure. Prior to administering preprocedural sedation, the operator should ascertain that informed consent has been obtained and that all of the patient's questions have been answered.

The objective of preprocedural sedation is to maximize procedure safety by making the patient cooperative, calm, and relaxed. The goal should be to achieve **conscious sedation: a state where the patient has a depressed level of consciousness but still maintains the independent ability to preserve a patent airway and respond appropriately and quickly to verbal and/or physical stimuli.** Prior to administration of preprocedural seda-

TABLE 2-1. COMMONLY USED DOSES OF PREPROCEDURAL SEDATION MEDICATIONS

Medication	Oral Dose	I.V. Dose	Comments
Benzodiazepines			
Diazepam (Valium)	5–10 mg	2–5 mg	—
Lorazepam	0.5–2 mg	1–2 mg	—
Midazolam (Versed)	N/A	0.5–2 mg	—
Opioids			
Fentanyl	N/A	25–50 μg	—
Morphine	15–30 mg	1–4 mg	—
Meperidine (Demerol)	50–150 mg	50–100 mg	—
Antihistamines			
Diphenhydramine (Benadryl)	25–50 mg	25–50 mg	—
Promethazine hydrochloride (Phenergan)	25–50 mg	12.5–25 mg	—
Antagonists			
Naloxone (Narcan)	N/A	0.4–2 mg	Repeat dose q2–3min to achieve effect or to a maximum dose of 10 mg
Flumazenil (Romazicon)	N/A	0.2 mg over 15 sec	Repeat dose q1min to achieve effect or to a maximum dose of 3 mg

I.V., intravenous; N/A, not applicable.

tion, the operator should examine the patient with special attention to the airway to identify patients who may require additional caution when using sedative agents (e.g., problems with sleep apnea, laryngeal mass, intrinsic pulmonary disease).

Factors that may influence the selection and dose of sedative include the patient's age and weight, level of anxiety, pain threshold, drug allergies, comorbid medical illnesses, potential drug interactions, and anticipated length of procedure. If preprocedural sedation is initiated with oral medications, they should be administered at least 1 hour prior to the patient's arrival at the catheterization laboratory. Table 2-1 lists commonly used medications for preprocedural sedation and their antagonists. A benzodiazepine is usually the initial drug of choice since it is not only a sedative and anxiolytic, but also achieves a limited degree of retrograde amnesia. Midazolam (Versed) is often the preferred benzodiazepine because of its rapid onset of action and relative short duration of effect. Initial doses range from 0.5 to 2 mg i.v., which may be repeated every few minutes until desired sedation is achieved. If further sedation is needed, administering a short-acting opioid such as fentanyl (25 to 50 µg) often results in adequate patient comfort.

CONTRAST AGENTS

Overview of Available Contrast Agents

All intravascular contrast agents contain iodine, which absorbs x-rays to a greater degree than surrounding tissue, and allows for intravascular opacification. Contrast agents are commonly classified based on their osmolality (high, low, or isosmolar) and their ionicity (ionic or nonionic). High-osmolar agents are ionic and are differentiated by whether or not they possess calcium-binding properties. Low-osmolar agents are classified by their ionicity. Ionic agents have six iodine atoms associated with two osmotically active particles, thus resulting in an osmolality that is six to seven times greater than serum osmolality. In contrast, nonionic agents have three iodine atoms for each osmotically active particle, resulting in an osmolality roughly 66% less than that of ionic agents and roughly twice that of serum osmolality. Table 2-2 lists examples of the commonly used contrast agents used in coronary angiography.

Adverse Effects

Many of the studies that have attempted to differentiate between the various adverse effects of contrast agents have been contradictory, making it difficult to make firm recommendations for use of a particular agent. Selection of a particular agent varies among insti-

TABLE 2-2. CONTRAST AGENTS

Class	Generic Name	Trade Name	Iodine (mg/mL)	Osmolality (mOsm/kg H_2O)	Viscosity (37°F)	Sodium Content (mEq/L)	Additives
Ionic							
High osmolar	Diatrizoate	Renografin-76	370	1,940	8.4	190	Sodium citrate, disodium EDTA
		Hypaque-76	370	2,076	8.32	160	Calcium disodium EDTA
		MD 76 R	370	2,140	9.1	190	Sodium citrate, disodium EDTA
		Angiovist 370	370	2,076	8.4	150	Calcium disodium EDTA
Low osmolar	Ioxaglate	Hexabrix	320	600	7.5	157	Calcium disodium EDTA
Nonionic							
Low osmolar	Iohexol	Omnipaque	350	844	10.4	Trace	Tromethamine, calcium disodium EDTA
	Iopamidol	Isovue 370	370	796	9.4	Trace	Tromethamine, calcium disodium EDTA
	Ioversol	Optiray 320	320	702	5.8	Trace	Tromethamine, calcium disodium EDTA
	Ioxilan	Oxilan 350	350	695	8.1	Trace	Citric acid, edetate calcium disodium
Isosmolar	Iodixanol	Visipaque 320	320	290	11.8	Trace	Tromethamine, edetate calcium disodium, calcium chloride dihydrate, sodium chloride

EDTA, ethylenediaminetetraacetate.

tutions and operators, and is often made based on personal experience and preference. Some basic guidelines regarding choice of agent will be presented in the following sections.

Effect on Myocardial Function

The physiological and adverse effects of contrast agents on myocardial and electrophysiological function are governed largely by three properties of contrast agents: osmolality, sodium concentration, and calcium-binding ability. The degree of myocardial depression, peripheral vasodilation, and elevation of left ventricular filling pressures seen with contrast agents is more marked with agents that have higher osmolality, are more hypertonic with respect to sodium, and have calcium-binding properties. This is even more apparent when larger boluses of contrast agents are used during ventriculography or aortography. In these settings, it is not uncommon to have peripheral vasodilation with a transient reduction in systolic blood pressure of 20 to 50 mm Hg and corresponding compensatory increase in heart rate with the use of high-osmolar agents. **These hemodynamic perturbations can be particularly catastrophic in patients with relatively low cardiac reserve such as left main coronary artery disease, severe aortic stenosis, or severe left ventricular dysfunction (See Chapter 7).** In contrast, low-osmolality agents typically cause a reduction in systolic blood pressure of only 5 to 15 mm Hg, with no change in heart rate during ventriculography or aortography.

Electrophysiologic and Electrocardiographic Effects

Electrocardiographic changes such as widening of the QRS complex, ST-segment changes, and prolongation of the QT interval are much less dramatic with the use of nonionic contrast agents. However, studies have shown that there is **no major difference in the incidence of ventricular or other tachyarrhythmias or ventricular fibrillation (range 0.1–1%) with the use of different contrast agents.** Furthermore, there appears to be no major difference in the incidence of ventricular fibrillation among contrast agents (range, 0.1% to 1%). With the intracoronary injection of contrast, one can often provoke transient sinus bradycardia or even sinus arrest. This usually occurs within a few seconds after injection, reaches peak effect after about 5 to 10 seconds, and resolves generally within 30 to 60 seconds. Possible explanations for this phenomenon include direct alteration of sinoatrial node function or provocation of the Bezold–Jarisch reflex. Depression of the atrioventricular node also occurs with the injection of intracoronary contrast agents via similar mechanisms. **Bradyarrhythmias occur less frequently with the use of low-osmolar, nonionic agents**.

Effect on Coagulation

It appears from *in vitro* and clinical studies that nonionic contrast agents are more prothrombotic than ionic agents. Whether or not this is clinically significant is controversial. However, some cardiac catheterization laboratories add heparin 5 IU/mL to nonionic contrast to avoid thrombosis.

Effect on Renal Function

Various factors (Table 2-3) may predispose a patient to deterioration in renal function. The exact mechanism remains unknown; possible explanations include renovascular vasoconstriction, changes in glomerular permeability, direct tubular injury, and tubular obstruction. **Contrast-induced renal dysfunction is usually evident within the first 48 hours, peaks within the first 5 days after the catheterization, and gradually returns to baseline function within 10 days.** Less than 1% of patients who suffer from contrast-induced renal dysfunction ultimately require chronic dialysis.

Limiting contrast volume for all patients to less than 3 mL/kg may be beneficial in reducing the incidence of postprocedural renal failure. For patients with chronic renal insufficiency, use of as little contrast as possible (less than 30 mL, if possible) appears to be related to a reduction in subsequent dialysis. Although animal studies have suggested that nonionic and/or low-osmolality agents may be associated with less contrast-induced renal failure, large-scale randomized, prospective human clinical trials have failed to show a consistent benefit with these agents in comparison to their ionic, high-osmolar counterparts. However, it is reasonable to select a nonionic agent for patients with preexisting renal insufficiency (serum creatinine greater than 2.0 mg/dL or greater than 1.5 mg/dL among diabetics) who require coronary angiography. **Hydration with either normal saline or 0.45%**

TABLE 2-3. **RISK FACTORS FOR CONTRAST-INDUCED NEPHROPATHY**

Preexisting renal insufficiency
Diabetes mellitus
Hypovolemia
Congestive heart failure
High contrast volumes (>3 mL/kg)
Multiple myeloma
Female sex

TABLE 2-4. CONTRAST REACTIONS: PRESENTATION AND TREATMENT

Severity	Presentation	Onset	Treatment
Mild	Mild nausea, flushing, bradycardia, urticaria without hives or tongue swelling, transient bradycardia or vasovagal episodes	Within minutes of exposure	Usually self-limited. Supportive treatment usually includes observation and/or diphenhydramine 25–50 mg p.o. Atropine (0.5–1.0 mg i.v.) occasionally required
Moderate	Persistent nausea with vomiting, anaphylactoid reaction (urticaria with hives and tongue swelling), persistent symptomatic bradycardia or vasovagal episodes	Within minutes to hours of exposure	Usually requires treatment consisting of i.v. hydration, antihistamines (diphenhydramine 50 mg i.v. and famotidine 20 mg i.v.), steroids (e.g., hydrocortisone 100 mg i.v.), antiemetics (e.g., prochlorperazine 2 mg i.v.), and, for persistent bradycardia and/or vasovagal episodes, consider atropine (0.5–2.0 mg iv.). For anaphylactoid reactions, consider epinephrine (0.1–0.5 mg s.q. or i.m.; may repeat dose every 10–15 min)
Severe	Anaphylactic (bronchospasm, laryngeal edema, and hypotension)	Can occur immediately after a single dose of contrast	Life threatening and requires immediate and aggressive treatment. Epinephrine [1 mL of 1:10,000 solution (0.1 mg/mL)] i.v. q1min p.r.n., steroids (e.g., hydrocortisone 100 mg i.v.), antihistamines (diphenhydramine 50 mg i.v. and famotidine 20 mg i.v.), and rapid i.v. fluid expansion. Consider intubation if airway is compromised

i.v., intravenous; p.r.n., as needed; s.q., subcutaneously.

saline for 6 to 12 hours before and 12 to 24 hours after the procedure is critical to prevent contrast-induced renal failure. Use of acetylcysteine (Mucomyst) in high-risk patients (serum creatinine greater than 2.0 mg/dL) has also been associated with a reduced incidence of renal dysfunction in small studies using two doses of 600 mg for 2 days (starting the day prior to the procedure).

Contrast Reactions

Patients may have contrast reactions as mild as flushing or as severe as hemodynamic collapse secondary to an anaphylactoid reaction indistinguishable from anaphylaxis (Table 2-4).

The majority of reactions are not mediated by immunoglobin E, thus **are not truly allergic**. Regardless of their mechanism, the risk of a reaction to contrast is increased by 2 to 3 times in patients with a strong history of allergy or atopy such as asthma. Patients with allergies to seafood have a similar risk of an allergic reaction to contrast. Although patients with a previous contrast reaction are at increased risk of having a repeat adverse reaction, **repeat reactions are relatively rare, occurring only in 15% to 40% of patients who are reexposed to contrast agents.**

TROUBLESHOOTING

Managing Patients with a History of Prior Contrast Reactions

Patients with a prior reaction to contrast agents or a history of past anaphylactoid reaction should be premedicated with steroids (prednisone 40 mg p.o. q6h for four doses or hydrocortisone 100 mg i.v. at least 6 hours prior to the procedure) and antihistamines such as diphenhydramine (Benadryl) 50 mg i.v. or p.o. Patients with a past life-threatening reaction to contrast should be given a small amount of contrast agent (1 to 2 mL) and observed for a few minutes prior to proceeding with angiography. The use of nonionic contrast is associated with less nausea, vomiting, and mild urticaria, thus making it the contrast agent of choice for patients with a prior history of contrast reaction.

Cost

Nonionic, low-osmolar contrast agents are substantially more expensive (up to 10 to 25 times) than ionic, high-osmolar agents.

TABLE 2-5. SUGGESTED INDICATIONS FOR USING LOW-OSMOLAR CONTRAST

Severe coronary artery disease (left main or triple vessel disease)
Severe valvular disease, particularly aortic stenosis
Acute ischemia
History of previous contrast allergy
Severe bradycardia
Preexisting renal insufficiency (serum creatinine >2 mg/dL)
Diabetes mellitus (serum creatinine >1.5 mg/dL)
Hypovolemia
Moderate to severe left ventricular dysfunction
Hemodynamic instability
Painful angiography (i.e., internal mammary artery)

Summary and Guidelines for Selection of Contrast Agent

For the routine cardiac catheterization patient, an ionic, high-osmolar contrast remains the agent of choice, given its low cost and overall acceptable tolerability. However, in certain situations, a low osmotic, nonionic contrast should be considered (Table 2-5). **Regardless of the choice of contrast agent, the operator must remain alert for possible contrast reactions.**

RADIATION SAFETY

The main principle regarding radiation safety in cardiology is to keep the patient's and operator's exposure to a level as low as reasonably achievable (ALARA). The principle of ALARA is achieved by learning the various techniques for reducing radiation exposure and their possible effects on image quality (Table 2-6). If these techniques are not learned, operator and/or patient exposure to radiation may result in direct tissue injury (deterministic effects) and/or neoplasms and heritable alterations in reproductive cells (stochastic effects).

Operators should wear radiation dosimeter badges whenever they are working with a source of radiation. They should be worn at collar level either on the apron or attached to the thyroid shield. These badges are monitored at periodic intervals (usually monthly). **The annual effective whole-body dose limit for occupational radiation workers is 5 rem/yr (50 mGy/yr).**

The main source of radiation exposure for the operator is scatter from the patient. A secondary, less significant source is escape of x-rays through the shielding of the x-ray tube. Protection for the operator consists of shielding, proper positioning from the radiation source, and adjusting the fluoroscopic controls in an attempt to minimize radiation exposure while maintaining a high-quality image.

Personal shielding involves lead aprons, thyroid collars, and lead glasses. **Lead aprons should have shielding properties equiv-**

TABLE 2-6. RADIATION SAFETY PRINCIPLES AND CORRESPONDING EFFECTS ON IMAGE QUALITY

Method of Protection	Operator Exposure to Radiation	Patient Exposure to Radiation	Image Quality
Patient and Operator Protection			
Lead gown, thyroid collar	Reduced	Unchanged	Unchanged
Leaded glasses	Reduced	Unchanged	Unchanged
Lead shield above/below table	Reduced	Unchanged	Unchanged
Greater distance between operator and table	Reduced	Unchanged	Unchanged
Femoral vs brachial approach	Reduced	Unchanged	Unchanged
Operator's fingers out of radiation beam	Reduced	Unchanged	Unchanged
Move patient's arm out of field	Reduced	Reduced	Improved
Radiation Dose Reduction			
Shorter fluoroscopy, cine times	Reduced	Reduced	Unchanged
Pulsed fluoroscopy	Reduced	Reduced	Unchanged
Fewer pulses per second	Reduced	Reduced	Worse
Fewer cine frames per second	Reduced	Reduced	Worse
Greater distance between source and patient	Variable	Reduced	Improved
Less distance between image intensifier and patient	Reduced	Reduced	Improved
Electronic image magnification	Variable	Higher	Improved
Smaller collimator opening	Variable	Variable	Improved
Cranial, caudal angulation	Higher	Higher	Worse
Large patient, pleural effusion	Higher	Higher	Worse

alent to 0.5 mm of lead, which shields the covered areas of the operator from roughly 90% of scatter radiation. Lead glasses protect the operator from possible radiation-induced cataracts and should have side shields to decrease exposure to radiation from the lateral direction. Thyroid shields prevent exposure to large cumulative doses of radiation, which could lead to thyroid cancer. These items should be checked annually with fluoroscopy to inspect for possible cracks, holes, and other signs of deterioration. The catheterization table will commonly have two lead shields: one is a table side drape that protects the lower body of the operator; the other is an adjustable lead acrylic shield suspended from the ceiling to aid in the protection of the operator's head and upper torso.

The inverse square law addresses the important concept that radiation dose drops rapidly by the inverse square of the relative increase of distance from the radiation source. Operators can decrease their radiation exposure by taking a step back from the irradiated area before engaging in fluoroscopy. Moving the image intensifier (which is located above the patient) to as close to the patient as possible also reduces scatter radiation by reducing geometric magnification (radiation dose usually increases with the square of the magnification). Placing hands in the direct beam of radiation should only be done in cases of emergency.

Modifying fluoroscopic controls can also decrease radiation exposure for both the operator and patient; however, these modifications may occasionally reduce image quality. One of the "golden rules" for minimizing radiation exposure is **keeping beam-on time to an absolute minimum.** Fluoroscopy or cineangiography should not be engaged if the image on the monitor is not being used. Most fluoroscopic machines have an option that allows the operator to select the level of image quality (low, normal, high). Low-image quality reduces radiation dose rate, but often produces a snowy or noisy image. These images may be acceptable in certain situations such as checking position of a guidewire or catheter. Most fluoroscopic machines have pulsed fluoroscopy, which results in x-rays being produced in short bursts instead of a continuous stream as in conventional fluoroscopy. Reducing the pulse frequency to 15 or 7.5 pulses of x-rays per second will reduce radiation exposure at the cost of producing a somewhat flickering, choppy image. A similar result is seen when one reduces the cine frame rate. Applying collimators (blades outside the x-ray tube that block x-rays) to the area of interest not only reduces scatter radiation to the operator, but is also improves image quality.

Electronic magnification (field-of-view) size for image intensifiers consists of usually at least three magnifications: 9 in. (23 cm), 7 in. (17 cm), and 5 in. (13 cm). In general, the least magnification reduces the dose rate to the patient's skin. For example, without changing collimators, changing the field of view from 7 in. to 5 in. results in roughly a doubling in entrance dose to the patient's skin, with greater spatial resolution that may be important in evaluating small coronary arteries. The effect of increasing magnification on radiation dose rates for the operator and other personnel is variable since it depends on the relative changes in tube current and kilovoltage.

Increasing the distance between the x-ray source (located beneath the patient) and the patient also results in improved image quality and a reduction in entry dose to the patient's skin. Federal regulations dictate that a spacer be placed on the x-ray tube to maintain a minimum distance of 38 cm between the x-ray source and patient.

NEEDLE, WIRE, SHEATH, CATHETER SELECTION

Access Needle

Access needles typically consist of two types: an open-bore needle and a Seldinger-type needle, which has a stylet in place. Open-bore needles are easier to manage since they signal immediate blood return when the vessel of interest is punctured. However, they may have to be flushed periodically if repeated attempts at access are needed because they can become clogged with subcutaneous tissue, fat, or blood. The stylet in the Seldinger-type needle prevents blockage of the lumen of the needle with tissue or blood and is removed once the operator believes puncture of the artery has occurred.

Most needles are a standard length of between 2.75 to 3 in. A 1.5-in. 21- or 22-gauge (micropuncture) needle is commonly used for the percutaneous radial approach. They are conventionally sized by their outer diameter, which corresponds to an arbitrary gauging system. An increasing gauge number corresponds to a smaller diameter. Typically, an 18-gauge needle is used for the femoral or brachial approach, and a micropuncture kit containing a 22-gauge needle is used for the radial approach. When attempting access for left heart catheterization, the needle should be held at its hub so that the operator can feel arterial pulsations transmitted from the tip of the needle. Feeling these pulsations aids in guiding the operator to successful cannulation into the arterial circulation.

Guidewire

Once access is obtained, a guidewire is inserted into the needle prior to withdrawal of the needle and placement of an arterial sheath over the guidewire. Guidewires are also used to facilitate passage of diagnostic coronary catheters to the central aorta. The choice of guidewire should be made prior to obtaining arterial access. Most guidewires consist of three major components: a central core (commonly stainless steel or nitinol), distal flexible spring coil (usually platinum or tungsten), and an outer coating to decrease friction (silicon, Teflon, or other hydrophilic coating). If a patient has severely tortuous or atherosclerotic vessels, a flexible wire such as a Wholey can be used. Alternatively, a Glidewire (SCIMED, Edmonton, Alberta, Canada) may be of particular benefit because of its smooth hydrophilic coating and excellent torque control. Guidewire length varies among different manufacturers, but generally consist of three major types. Short wires (30 to 45 cm) are used in placing sheaths. Medium-length wires (125 to 150 cm) enable the operator to guide the diagnostic coronary catheter to the aorta. Long-length wires (250 to 300 cm) are employed when the operator wishes to exchange diagnostic coronary catheters without moving the wire tip (also refered to as an exchange wire). Wire tips are universally flexible, and are either straight or J tipped. **For the majority of cases, the J-tipped wire is preferred because it is less likely to induce vessel dissection and avoids entering small vessel branches.**

A straight-tipped wire is used mainly in attempting to cross a severely stenotic aortic valve or in obtaining brachial or radial arterial access.

Guidewire diameters also vary widely. The smaller-diameter guidewires (0.018 in., 0.021 in., 0.025 in.) are generally used with a Swan–Ganz catheter to augment stiffness. The 0.025-in. guidewire is also used in obtaining radial arterial access. The 0.032-in. guidewire is used mostly in brachial arterial access and intraaortic balloon placement. The most commonly used guidewires are the 0.035-in. and 0.038-in., used during most routine diagnostic left heart catheterizations. The 0.035-in. wire is usually preferred because it is more flexible and softer, thus less likely to cause a dissection. The 0.038-in. wire is used when increased stiffness is desired, such as when attempting dilator placement through calcified arteries or fibrotic tissue. Larger-diameter guidewires are used predominantly in interventional cases where larger sheaths and catheter sizes are often necessary.

Dilators and Sheaths

Vascular sheaths generally contain a removable dilator, a diaphragm that prevents leakage of blood or air into the sheath, and a sidearm connected to a three-way stopcock, which allows the operator to record pressure measurements, flush the sheath, and infuse medications. The dilator is made of stiff plastic (usually Teflon or polyethylene) that allows it to pass through fibrous subcutaneous tissue or atherosclerotic/calcified vessels. Generally, the sheaths used range from 5 to 8F[a] catheter, although larger-sized sheaths are sometimes used in interventional cases. For femoral and brachial diagnostic left heart catheterizations, 6F and 5F catheter sheaths, respectively, are most commonly used. For radial cases, a 4F or 5F catheter dilator is frequently used prior to insertion of either a 5F or 6F catheter sheath. In cases of severe peripheral vascular disease, a smaller dilator may need to be used initially prior to inserting a 5F or 6F catheter system.

The length of sheaths used routinely varies from 6 to 35 cm. For most cases, an 11-cm sheath is adequate. **Longer sheaths of 25 to 35 cm are selected when one encounters tortuous femoral and/or iliac arteries to facilitate torque control of the diagnostic coronary catheter.** Occasionally, with the radial approach, a longer 23-cm sheath is used to prevent radial artery spasm.

---

[a]F, French scale. Used to denote the size of tubular instruments such as catheters and sounds. One F is roughly equivalent to 0.33 mm in diameter.

CATHETER SELECTION

As discussed in Chapter 1, the operator should review, if available, any past coronary angiographic films to observe the catheters used for diagnostic cardiac angiography and to identify possible difficulties encountered when the native coronary arteries and/or bypass grafts were engaged.

The sections of an angiographic catheter include a body (which is mostly straight throughout its course) and the tip, with various curves. The curves are classified as primary, secondary, and tertiary starting from the tip (Figure 2-1). The hub of the catheter has an airtight seal composed of a female Luer–Lok that allows attachment to a syringe or manifold, winged tips to facilitate catheter rotation, and labeling of the size of the catheter.

Diagnostic coronary catheters are sized by their external diameter. Most diagnostic coronary catheterizations will use 6F catheters, although catheters as small as 4F and as large as 8F may occasionally be used. Catheter length varies based on the percutaneous approach and their configuration. Most pigtail catheters for ventriculography or aortography are 110 cm in length, while the commonly used Judkins catheters for coronary angiography are 100 cm in length. Brachial catheters are generally 80 or 100 cm long.

Catheter selection depends on the percutaneous approach used, whether bypass grafts are present, and on coronary anatomy variations. For the left femoral, left brachial, and left radial approach, the Judkins catheters are usually the initial catheters selected. Both the left and right Judkins catheters have a primary curve of 90 degrees. The left Judkins (JL) has a secondary curve of 180 degrees, while the right Judkins (JR) has a secondary curve of 30 degrees. The JL catheter comes in various arm (distance between the primary and secondary curve) sizes. For example, the JL4 catheter has an arm length of 4.2 cm, and the JL5 and JL6 catheters have arm lengths of 5.2 cm and 6.2 cm, respectively. For most diagnostic cases, the JL4 catheter is used first. If the patient's aortic root is dilated, then a longer-arm JL catheter (JL5 or JL6) is frequently used. A smaller-arm (JL3.5) catheter is chosen if the aortic root is smaller than usual or if the left main is located superiorly. In cases where a short left main trunk is encountered, a JL4 short-tip catheter usually successfully cannulates the left main ostium. If one is unable to engage the left coronary circulation with the Judkins catheters, the left Amplatz (AL) class of catheters is usually employed.

The AL catheters are particularly good at engaging a short left main trunk or in cases where the left circumflex coronary artery

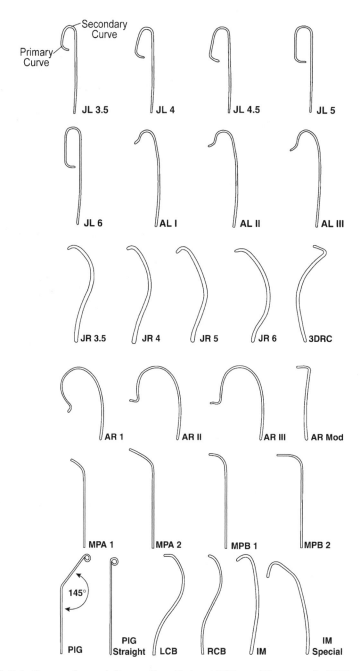

FIG. 2-1. Commonly used diagnostic catheters. *MPA*, multipurpose A; *MPB*, multipurpose B; *PIG*, pigtail; *LCB*, left coronary bypass; *RCB*, right coronary bypass; *IM*, internal mammary; *JR*, Judkins right; *AR*, Amplatz right; *AR Mod*, Amplatz right modified; *JL*, Judkins left; *AL*, Amplatz left.

(LCX) and left anterior descending coronary artery (LAD) have separate ostia. They can also be used to engage high-anterior right coronary arteries (RCAs) or Shepherd's Crook RCA. The right Amplatz (AR) catheters are useful for cannulating RCAs that have an inferior orientation. Amplatz catheters are classified by the size of their secondary curve (AL1 to 3; AR1 to 3). Alternatively, a 3DRC (No Torque Right) catheter (Cordis Corp., Miami, FL, U.S.A.) can be attempted in cases where the RCA ostium cannot be engaged with the JR4. The three-dimensional curve configuration of the 3DRC catheter facilitates engagement of the RCA.

For the right arm approach (either brachial or radial), either the Amplatz, multipurpose, or modified brachial catheters are commonly used. One advantage of the multipurpose catheter is its ability to be used for both coronary angiography and ventriculography. The multipurpose catheter can also be used from the femoral approach, usually in cases where the RCA or left main have an inferior takeoff. Both the multipurpose and Amplatz catheters require experience for proper manipulation. **To minimize risk of coronary dissection when using the Amplatz catheters, the operator should rotate the catheter counterclockwise to disengage it from the coronary ostium prior to removing the catheter.**

For bypass grafts, the JR4 catheter is usually successful in engaging both venous and arterial grafts. For left internal mammary artery (LIMA) or right internal mammary artery (RIMA) grafts that have a sharply angulated downward takeoff, the IMA catheter is more likely to successfully engage these grafts since it has a longer tip and less of a primary curve (80 degrees) than the JR4. The JoMed (JoMed, Alpharetta, GA, U.S.A.) 5F catheter is stiffer and more angulated than the IMA catheter and may be used for engaging a LIMA graft that has a sharp, downward takeoff. However, the JR4 is usually used first to engage the subclavian artery, and a long J-wire is used to exchange the JR4 for the IMA catheter. For saphenous vein grafts (SVG) to RCA grafts that have a steep downward orientation, the multipurpose, right-bypass, or right-modified Amplatz catheters can be attempted if the JR4 approach is unsuccessful. Whenever SVGs to the LAD or LCX cannot be cannulated with a JR4, alternative catheters such as the left bypass, AL, or multipurpose can be considered.

MANIFOLD

A variety of manifold systems exist. One common design is a three-component manifold that has three stopcocks attached. The first stopcock is connected to a pressure transducer, the second is attached to flush solution, and the third is attached to the contrast agent of choice. When setting up the manifold, it is vital to ensure that the pressure transducer tubing is flushed adequately with saline to prevent any air bubbles from interfering with pressure measurements. Shorter and stiffer tubing between the pressure transducer and catheter optimize pressure measurements. The pressure transducer is "zeroed" with the aid of an assistant by placing the transducer at the patient's mid-chest level. The stopcock to the saline port is then opened to bring down the saline through the connection tubing into the manifold. Similarly, the stopcock to the contrast agent of choice is opened and the contrast is brought down to the stopcock level. The manifold is then once again flushed with saline and all tubing is inspected for air bubbles.

PERCUTANEOUS VASCULAR ACCESS
Femoral Approach

The femoral approach is the most common in the United States. The operator should first identify anatomical landmarks prior to giving local anesthesia, such as the inguinal ligament, which traverses from the anterior superior iliac spine to the pubic tubercle. The femoral artery generally crosses the inguinal ligament at an imaginary point that is located one-third from the medial aspect and two thirds from the lateral aspect of the ligament. The femoral pulse is then palpated approximately two finger breadths (2 to 3 cm) below the inguinal ligament, marking the site of arterial access (Figure 2-2). One can also use fluoroscopy to identify the femoral head. The optimal access location would be at the site over the inferior border of the femoral head. This approach is especially useful in obese patients where the identification of the inguinal ligament may be more difficult. Approximately 95% of patients have the femoral bifurcation located below the upper border of the femoral head. **Locating the optimal site of entry is important. Entry sites above the inguinal ligament may lead to an increased risk of retroperitoneal bleeding, while entry sites that are too low may result in the development of arteriovenous fistula or pseudoaneurysm.**

After the entry site is determined, the femoral region is scrubbed with povidone–iodine (Betadine) and surgically draped. The entry site is again palpated with the index and middle fingers of the left hand, either perpendicular or parallel to the artery, to confirm location of the femoral pulse. With the left index and middle fingers maintaining constant moderate pressure on the artery, the operator uses their right hand to raise a subcutaneous wheal at the entry site with a 25-gauge needle containing roughly 3 mL of procaine 1%. A 22-gauge needle is

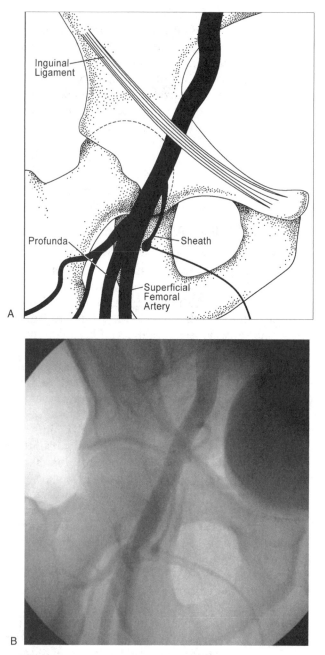

FIG. 2-2. Femoral access landmarks. **A:** Diagram of femoral artery landmarks. **B:** Thirty-degree left anterior oblique (LAO) coronary artery projection of the femoral artery. The LAO best displays the bifurcation of the profunda and superficial femoral artery.

then used to slowly deliver an additional 6 to 10 mL of local anesthetic to the deeper subcutaneous tissue. The amount of local anesthetic should cover the anticipated needle path from the skin to the artery. When giving local anesthesia, the operator should monitor the ECG and the patient for any signs of a possible vagal reaction.

TROUBLESHOOTING

The patient is allergic to procaine: If the patient has a documented allergy to procaine (ester prototype anesthetics), then lidocaine 2% or other amide prototype local anesthetic can be given.

Holding the 18-gauge Cook (Cook, Inc.) access needle at the hub with the thumb and index finger, the operator inserts the needle through the skin at a 30- to 45-degree angle with the bevel pointed upwards. As the needle nears the femoral artery, the operator should observe the motion of the needle. A side-to-side motion usually signals that the needle is either lateral or medial to the artery, and should be repositioned. If the needle motion is up-and-down, the needle is positioned correctly, and the needle should be gently advanced. As the needle gets closer to the artery, the operator may feel arterial pulsations transmitted through the needle hub. Brisk, pulsatile blood return signals successful arterial puncture. A 45-cm J-tipped 0.035-cm guidewire is then advanced through the needle. The needle is removed, and a small nick is made at the level of the skin with a scalpel to facilitate insertion of the sheath size of choice (usually 6F catheter) over the guidewire. The dilator within the sheath and the guidewire are subsequently removed, along with the sheath flushed with saline. The arterial pressure should then be documented by attaching the side port of the sheath to the manifold.

In cases of morbid obesity, severe peripheral vascular disease, aortic dissection, or aortic aneurysm, the femoral approach is either very difficult or contraindicated. If coronary angiography is indicated, the brachial or radial approaches should be used. Because the brachial and radial arteries are smaller caliber vessels, heparin (3,000 to 5,000 units i.v.) should be used to avoid arterial thrombosis.

Brachial Approach

Prior to local anesthesia, the brachial and radial pulses of both arms should be palpated. The Allen test should also be performed. The brachial artery is approximately 3 to 5 mm in diameter. The strongest brachial pulse is generally located 1 to 2 cm above the elbow crease. The antecubital fossa is then sterilized and draped. Using a 25-gauge needle, a small wheal is raised using approximately 3 mL of local anesthetic. Injecting larger amounts of local anesthetic may make it more difficult to palpate the brachial pulse. One can use either an 18- or 22-gauge (micropuncture) needle to obtain arterial access using a 45-degree angle. With the micropuncture needle kit, a stiffer 0.025-in. guidewire is used, and the standard 0.035-in. guidewire is used for the 18-gauge needle. Once the guidewire is inserted into the artery, a 5F or 6F catheter sheath is usually inserted as described in the percutaneous femoral approach. Heparin 3,000 to 5,000 units i.v. should be considered to avoid sheath thrombosis.

Radial Approach

As described with the brachial approach, the Allen test should be performed prior to radial artery catheterization. The left radial approach is generally preferred because it is less difficult to engage the coronary arteries than it is with the right radial approach. The patient's arm is abducted at a 70-degree angle and the wrist is hyperextended. Topical anesthetic cream is then applied over the radial artery to reduce the amount of local anesthetic needed after the area is cleaned in a sterile fashion and draped. Local anesthesia is then given as depicted in the brachial approach. Next, either an 18- or 22-gauge needle is inserted at a 30- to 45-degree angle approximately 1 cm from the styloid process. The guidewire is then advanced as described in the brachial approach. A 4F or 5F catheter dilator is then used to predilate the radial artery. A 5F catheter or 6F catheter sheath is then inserted over a standard 0.035-in. guidewire. A longer sheath (23 cm) may be used in radial cases to decrease radial artery spasm. Alternatively, standard sheath lengths may be used with local infusions of nitroglycerine or verapamil. Heparin 3,000 to 5,000 units i.v. should be considered to avoid sheath thrombosis.

TROUBLESHOOTING
Poor Blood Return

Weak blood flow may signal that the needle may be located against the vessel wall, subintimally, or in a smaller branch. Gentle forward or backward manipulation or a slight change in the angulation of the needle may improve blood flow. Alternatively, sluggish blood flow may be secondary to severe peripheral vascular disease or low perfusion states.

Resistance Advancing the Guidewire Is Encountered

The guidewire should only be inserted through the needle when brisk, pulsatile blood flow is obtained. If resistance is encountered as the guidewire is passing through the tip of the needle and it is not relieved by reducing the angle of the needle, the guidewire should be removed and brisk pulsatile blood flow should be confirmed. If blood flow is not brisk, the needle may be gently redirected in an attempt to restore blood flow. If these maneuvers are unsuccessful, the needle should be removed and pressure held over the entry site for 5 minutes before reattempting access. If resistance is encountered or the patient begins to complain of pain after the guidewire has been successfully advanced a few centimeters, fluoroscopy should be used to document location of the guidewire. In this situation, the needle is removed, and a small sheath (5F catheter) can be carefully advanced to the point where resistance was encountered. The wire is then removed and the sheath aspirated to confirm blood return and flushed. By injecting a small amount (5 mL) of either nonionic or diluted ionic contrast under fluoroscopy the operator can assess for arterial dissection, vessel tortuosity, or severe atherosclerosis.

A Retrograde Subintimal Dissection Is Found after Access Is Secured

Subintimal retrograde dissections caused by guidewire insertions rarely cause arterial complications. The patient should be monitored closely for signs and symptoms of dissection extension (progressive pain, pale extremities, loss of distal pulses). Either the other femoral artery, or a brachial or radial approach should be accessed for left heart catheterization.

Severe Vessel Tortuosity or Atherosclerosis Is Encountered

Reinserting the softer, more steerable Wholey guidewire or the hydrophilic-coated Glidewire may enable passage through the tortuosity or stenosis. A long sheath [45-cm Arrow (Arrow International, Reading, PA, U.S.A.) or 55-cm Brite Tip (Cordis Corp.) long sheath] should be considered to improve catheter manipulation.

Resistance During Sheath Placement Is Encountered

Confirm that an adequate nick has been made at the level of the skin. Resistance may also originate from severe vessel calcification or scar tissue from prior procedures. Using first a smaller dilator (4F or 5F catheter) to predilate along with a stiffer wire (0.038-cm or Amplatz wire) may facilitate placement of the sheath.

Femoral Pulse Is Not Easily Palpable

One could attempt using the Smart Needle (Escalon Vascular Access, Inc., New Berlin, WI, U.S.A.) device. With this device, the needle is directed to the site where the arterial pulsations are heard best via the Doppler probe.

Patient Has Prosthetic Femoral Artery Grafts

If the vascular graft is older than 2 to 3 months, the percutaneous femoral approach can be considered. Predilation with a smaller dilator is recommended prior to insertion of the desired sheath size to prevent the sheath from kinking when it passes through the graft.

SUGGESTED READINGS

Boucher RA, Myler RK, Clark DA, et al. Coronary angiography and angioplasty. *Catheter Cardiovasc Diagn* 1988;14:269–285.

Denys BG, Uretsky BF, Baughman K, et al.. Accessing vascular structures. In: Uretsky BF, ed. *Cardiac catheterization: concepts, techniques and applications.* Malden, MA: Blackwell Science, 1997:93–118.

Freed M, Grines C, Sagian RD, eds. *The new manual of interventional cardiology.* Birmingham, MI: Physicians' Press, 1997:1–64.

Limacher MC, Douglas PS, Germano G, et al. Radiation safety in the practice of cardiology. ACC expert consensus document. *J Am Coll Cardiol* 1998;31:892–913.

Mattai WH, Kussmal WG, Krol J, et al. A comparison of low- with high-osmolar contrast agent in cardiac angiography: identification of criteria for selective use. *Circulation* 1994;89:291–301.

Wagner LK, Archer BR. *Minimizing risks from fluoroscopic X-rays: bioeffects, instrumentation, and examination,* 3rd ed. Houston: Partners in Radiation Management, 2000.

3. NATIVE CORONARY ANGIOGRAPHY

Niranjan Seshadri, Robert E. Hobbs, and Sorin J. Brener

The coronary arteries arise from the sinuses of Valsalva. The left main coronary artery arises from the left sinus. After a short course, the left main trunk (LMT) usually bifurcates into the left anterior descending (LAD) and left circumflex (LCX) coronary arteries. In some instances, it may trifurcate, with the ramus intermedius being the intermediate vessel in the trifurcation. The current classification of coronary anatomy is based on the CASS (Coronary Artery Surgery Study) system.

The LAD follows a course along the anterior interventricular groove to the apex of the heart, supplying blood to the anterior wall, the septum via septal perforators, and the anterolateral wall via diagonal branches.

The LCX courses along the left atrioventricular groove, supplying the lateral wall of the left ventricle. The branches arising from the LCX are called obtuse marginals, with the first branch arising from the atrioventricular (AV) LCX called obtuse marginal 1, the second branch called obtuse marginal 2, and so forth.

The right coronary artery (RCA) arises from the right sinus of Valsalva and travels along the right AV groove. The first branch that arises from the RCA is the conus branch, which supplies the right ventricular outflow tract. In approximately 50% of the cases, the conus branch has a separate origin. Localizing the conus branch may be important in selected cases because it is often a critical source of collateral circulation to the LAD. Other branches include the artery to the sinus node, which arises from the RCA in 60% of cases; the acute marginal branches, which supply the right ventricle; the artery to the AV node; the diaphragmatic artery; and terminal branches [i.e., the posteroventricular branches and the posterior descending artery (PDA) in most cases].

The PDA, which courses along the posterior interventricular groove, determines coronary dominance. In 85% of the cases, the PDA arises from the RCA, making the coronary circulation right dominant. In 7% of the cases, the circulation is codominant, with the posterior interventricular groove being supplied by both the RCA and the LCX. In 8% of the cases, the PDA arises from the left circumflex, making it the dominant artery.

ENGAGING THE CORONARY ARTERIES

For diagnostic coronary angiography, we routinely use Judkins 6 French (F) left and right (JL6, JR6) catheters via the femoral approach. Use of smaller-caliber 4F or 5F catheter has some advantages. For example, in patients requiring only diagnostic angiography prior to heart valve surgery, use of a 4F catheter decreases recovery time and allows for faster ambulation after sheath removal (**See Chapter 8.**)

Engaging the Left Coronary Arteries

Assuming that the size of the aorta is within normal limits, a Judkins left 4F catheter (JL4) is routinely used. The catheters are flushed with heparinized saline and advanced over a J-tipped guidewire ("J wire") through the femoral sheath and to the ascending aorta just above the aortic root. **To avoid retrograde dissection of the aorta, catheters are advanced with the J-tipped guidewire protruding beyond the proximal end of the catheter.** Once the catheter is just above the sinus of Valsalva, the guidewire is withdrawn and a few drops of blood are allowed to back-bleed from the catheter, allowing for clearance of debris that may have collected during catheter advancement. The catheter is then connected to the manifold, flushed with saline, and the syringe is loaded with dye. Once an adequate pressure tracing is achieved, the catheter is opacified with 1 to 2 mL of contrast dye and is ready for selective engagement.

TROUBLESHOOTING
The Catheter Does Not Back-Bleed

If the catheter does not back-bleed after removing the guidewire, the tip may be apposed to the wall of the aorta. Gently withdraw the catheter, and turn it either clockwise or counterclockwise to free the catheter tip. After discarding a few drops of blood, connect the catheter hub to the manifold and look at the pressure tracing.

No Waveform is Observed in the Pressure Tracing

If no waveform is observed in the pressure tracing, the transducer may not be opened to pressure. This may be rectified by manipulating the first of the three-way stopcocks on the manifold or by turning the transducer at the side of the table to the "on" position.

Catheter is NOT Engaging and the Waveform is Damped

This may be due to air in the system or because the catheter may be partially against the arterial wall. To eliminate air from the system, first gently withdraw a few drops of blood and flush the manifold and catheter with saline, taking care not to reintroduce air into the system. A gentle clockwise or counterclockwise rotation, along with a pulling back of the catheter, will move the tip away from the aortic wall. If the damped waveform persists, it may be due to air in the pressure transducer tubing. Flush the transducer tubing and recheck the pressure. If the problem persists, in rare cases, the catheter itself may have a kink, in which case it needs to be replaced.

When using the Judkins technique, not much effort is required to cannulate the ostium of the LMT. The catheter is advanced into the aortic root and, in the majority of the patients, it will engage the ostium. The catheter tip should be coaxial with the LMT. In cases where the LMT is not easily cannulated, a clockwise or a counterclockwise rotation may help engage the ostium.

TROUBLESHOOTING

The Aorta is Dilated, and it is Difficult to Engage the LMT with the JL4

In cases of dilated aortas, the curve on the JL4 catheter may be too short to engage the ostium of the LMT. Upsizing to a JL5 or even JL6 catheter may help. Additionally, with dilated aortas there may not be a hinge point for the arm of the catheter to rest. In this case, a counterclockwise (moves the catheter anteriorly) or a clockwise (moves the catheter posteriorly) rotation helps engage the ostium.

The LMT Has an Unusual Takeoff

In some cases, the ostium of the LMT may have a takeoff (usually a high posterior origin) in a plane that may be out of reach of the Judkins catheters. Switching to an Amplatz system may be helpful. Amplatz catheters are advanced around the aortic arch over a guidewire. The catheter is further advanced until the curve rests in the left sinus of Valsalva, with the tip facing the ostium of the LMT. Withdrawal and gentle clockwise and/or counterclockwise rotation brings the tip in plane with the coronary ostia. To disengage the Amplatz catheter, push it gently forward (brings the tip out of the coronary ostium) and rotate before pulling back, all under fluoroscopic guidance.

Once the ostium of the LMT is engaged, a good pressure waveform should be visualized before proceeding with coronary arteriography.

TROUBLESHOOTING

The Ostium is Engaged and the Waveform is damped

A damped pressure waveform (drop in the catheter-tip systolic pressure) or a ventricularized pressure waveform (drop in the catheter-tip diastolic pressure) usually indicates that the catheter tip is either deep-seated, thereby restricting coronary inflow, or that the tip is against the wall. It also indicates the possibility of significant left main stenosis. The catheter tip should be immediately withdrawn from the ostium. The ostium can be reengaged cautiously. If a small injection of dye reveals significant ostial left main stenosis (another clue may be the absence of dye reflux into the aortic root with the injection), two short cine runs aimed at visualizing distal targets for bypass surgery should promptly be performed, with the catheter then immediately pulled back from the ostium. Care must be taken to avoid multiple engagements of the LMT, as this can lead to abrupt vessel closure. In cases where significant LMT stenosis is suspected, the operator can take nonselective angiograms of the LMT by injecting dye, with the catheter tip positioned in left sinus. Catheter damping may also be seen in cases of spasm of the LMT. In such instances, intracoronary nitroglycerin can be injected (200 µg) and a follow-up picture can be taken to document relief of spasm.

Engaging the Right Coronary Artery

The JR4 catheter is most commonly used to engage the right coronary ostium. The JR4 is advanced to the right coronary cusp, with the tip facing the left ostium. The catheter is gently pulled back while simultaneously rotated clockwise to engage the right ostium (the tip of the catheter tends to migrate down towards the sinuses with clockwise rotation). Alternatively, the clockwise rotation may be performed above the plane of the right coronary ostium without pulling back. This will make the catheter tip move down towards the sinus while rotating. After engaging, the pressure waveform is visualized and, if satisfactory, coronary arteriography may be performed. Troubleshooting, advancing, and engaging of the RCA is the same as for the left coronary artery.

TROUBLESHOOTING

Difficulty Engaging the RCA with the JR4

The ostium may be high and anterior, posterior, or angled upwardly. A 3DRC (Cordis Corp., Miami, FL, U.S.A.) catheter may be used if the JR4 catheter fails to engage the ostium. This catheter is dropped to the aortic valve and gently pulled back without rotating the catheter. For a high and anterior take off (frequently seen in transplanted hearts due to rotation of the heart), pulling the catheter further back with a less clockwise turn usually engages the ostium. For a posteriorly directed ostium, further clockwise rotation may be required. For an upwardly directed ostium or dilatated ascending aorta, an Amplatz catheter works well. To engage the ostium of the RCA arising from the left sinus of Valsalva, an Amplatz left (AL1) catheter may be used. Other catheters that may be used include an Amplatz right or a multipurpose catheter.

The Pressure Waveform is Damped or Ventricularized

This usually indicates the catheter tip is either deep-seated, thereby restricting coronary inflow, the tip is against the wall, or there may be spasm or severe disease of the ostium. If the catheter tip is too far in the artery, the catheter is withdrawn gently without disengaging the ostium, with a gentle counterclockwise rotation usually stabilizing the catheter. A gentle clockwise or counterclockwise rotation moves the tip away from the ostium. If spasm is suspected, a gentle test injection is performed. The catheter is disengaged, gently reengaged and intracoronary nitroglycerin or a sublingual nitroglycerin is administered, provided the blood pressure is acceptable and the image remains suspicious for spasm. If there is true ostial narrowing, a quick injection with just enough dye to fill the artery is administered and the catheter is removed from the ostium. Failure to promptly remove the catheter from the ostium of the artery, or proceeding with angiography in the presence of a damped waveform, may increase the risk of inducing ventricular fibrillation. Ostial spasm usually occurs a few seconds after engaging the artery. This helps differentiate it from a fixed stenosis.

CORONARY ANGIOGRAPHIC VIEWS

Coronary arteriography provides a silhouette of the epicardial coronary arteries. Several orthogonal views of each vessel are required to ensure a complete evaluation. The basic views, posteroanterior (PA), left anterior oblique (LAO), and right anterior oblique (RAO) with or without varying degrees of either cranial of caudal angulation, show the coronaries in orthogonal views while minimizing interference by other structures, such as the spine and the diaphragm.

In the LAO projection, the image intensifier (II) is to the left of the patient. On fluoroscopy, the spine is to the right of the screen in a LAO view. In the RAO projection, the II is to the right of the patient and the spine is on the left of the screen in fluoroscopy. In general, cranial angulation is ideal for visualizing the distal portion of vessels, and caudal angulation is ideal for visualizing the proximal portion of vessels. The commonly used views shown in Table 3-1 represent only a guide and should be modified for each individual patient.

During cine runs, patients should be instructed to take in a deep breath, especially with cranial angulations, to move the diaphragm out of view as far as possible.

Left Coronary Views

The first view of the left coronary system should delineate the course of the left main coronary trunk. Most operators prefer either a straight PA or a 20-degree RAO and 20-degree caudal angulation (Figure 3-1). The spine should be off the origin of the left main coronary trunk.

The 20-degree RAO, 20-degree caudal view is an ideal view for the proximal circumflex. In this view, while panning down the circum-

TABLE 3-1. COMMONLY USED ANGIOGRAPHIC VIEWS

Vessel Optimally Viewed	
Left coronary artery	
20 degrees RAO, 20 degrees caudal	LMT and LCX
40 degrees PA cranial	LAD
45 degrees LAO, 30 degrees cranial	LAD and diagonals
30 degrees RAO, 30 degrees cranial	LAD
45 degrees LAO, 30 degrees caudal	LMT, proximal LAD, proximal LCX, and collaterals to the RCA
Right coronary artery	
40 degrees LAO	Proximal and mid-RCA
40 degrees PA cranial	Distal RCA (PDA and PV branches)
35 degrees RAO	Proximal and mid-RCA

LAD, left anterior descending; LAO, left anterior oblique; LCX, left circumflex coronary artery; LMT, left main trunk; PA, posteroanterior; PDA, posterior descending artery; PV, pulmonary vascular; RAO, right anterior oblique; RCA, right coronary artery.

flex, portions of the LAD may also be visualized. The operator can also visualize the LCX by using a straight PA 30-degree caudal view.

A straight PA 40-degree cranial angulation view highlights the mid and distal portions of the LAD (Figure 3-2). To separate out the diagonals from the LAD, a 30-degree RAO with a 25- to 30-degree cranial angulation is used. The diagonals are placed above the LAD in this view. Another useful view to separate the diagonals from the LAD is the 40- to 50-degree LAO and 25- to 30-degree cranial views (Figure 3-3).

The proximal LAD and the left main coronary artery can also be visualized using the 45-degree LAO and 30-degree caudal view (Figure 3-4). This view is also known as the "spider view". The origins of the LCX and the proximal diagonals can also be seen well with this view.

In cases where the mid-LAD needs to be visualized in additional views, such as would be the case for LIMA graft insertions, the straight lateral view 90-degree LAO is very useful.

Right Coronary Views

The RCA is viewed in either a straight RAO or LAO (35 to 40 degrees) view (Figure 3-5) or a PA view with cranial angulation. The 40-degree LAO view shows the ostium, proximal, and mid portions best (Figure 3-6), but the PDA and the posteroventricular branches are also well visualized.

The bifurcation of the RCA, PDA and the posteroventricular branches are best seen in the 40-degree PA cranial view.

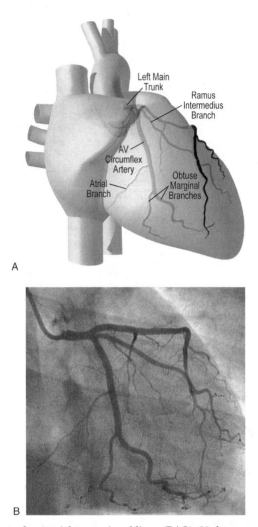

FIG. 3-1. Twenty-degree right anterior oblique (RAO), 20-degree caudal view of the left coronary artery. **A:** Three-dimensional diagram of the 20-degree RAO, 20-degree caudal view. **B:** Angiogram of the 20-degree RAO, 20-degree caudal view. This view is optimal for visualization of the left main trunk and left circumflex (LCX) arteries. Note that the LCX courses posterior to the heart in this view, a detail best appreciated in the three-dimensional diagram. As in all RAO views, the spine and the diagnostic catheter lie to the left of the heart.

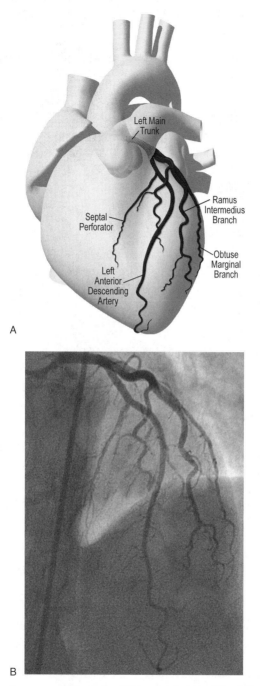

FIG. 3-2. Forty-degree posteroanterior (PA) cranial view of the left coronary artery. **A:** Three-dimensional diagram of the 40-degree PA cranial view. **B:** Angiogram of the 40-degree PA cranial view. This view is optimal for visualization of the mid and distal portion of the left anterior descending artery (LAD) and proximal portion of all diagonal branches.

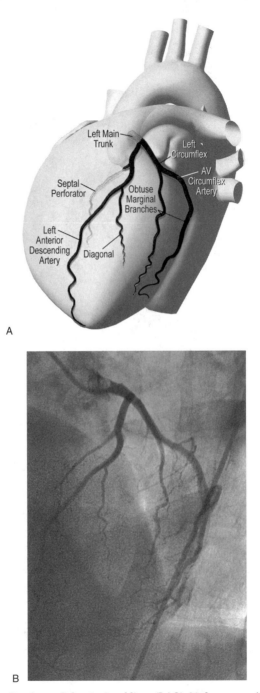

FIG. 3-3. Forty-five-degree left anterior oblique (LAO), 20-degree cranial view of the left coronary artery. **A:** Three-dimensional diagram of the 45-degree LAO, 20-degree cranial view. **B:** Angiogram of the 45-degree LAO, 20-degree cranial view. This view is optimal for visualization of the left anterior descending and the entire length of the diagonal branches. As in all LAO views, the catheter and the spine are to the right of the heart.

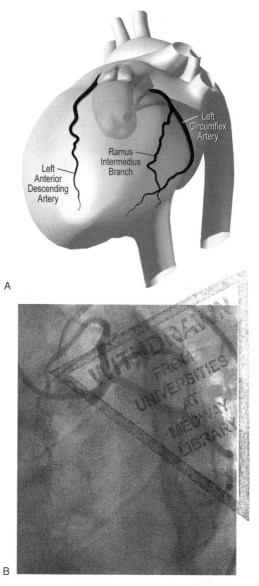

FIG. 3-4. Fifty-degree left anterior oblique (LAO), 35-degree caudal view of the left coronary artery ("spider view"). **A:** Three-dimensional diagram of the 50-degree LAO, 35-degree caudal view. **B:** Angiogram of the 50-degree, LAO–35-degree caudal view. This view is optimal for visualization of the left main trunk and the proximal portions of the left anterior descending and the left circumflex arteries. In cases of occlusion of the right coronary artery (RCA), it is important to maintain cine long enough to visualize the extent of potential collaterals to the RCA.

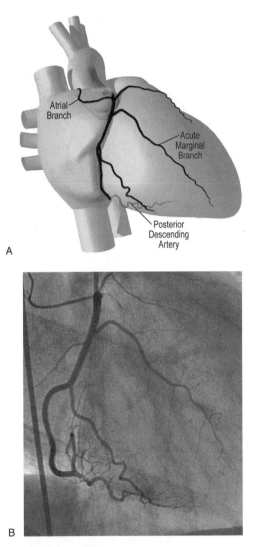

FIG. 3-5. Thirty-degree right anterior oblique view of the right coronary artery. **A:** Three-dimensional diagram of the 35-degree left anterior oblique (LAO) view. **B:** Angiogram of the 35-degree LAO view. This view is best for visualization of the posterior descending branch of the RCA.

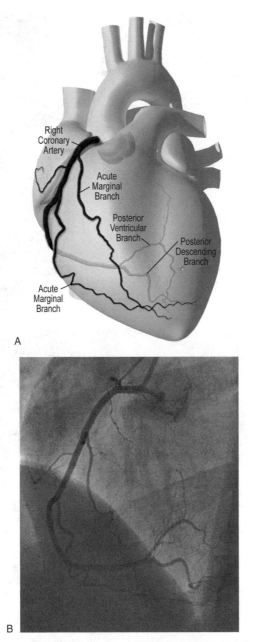

A

B

FIG. 3-6. Thirty-five-degree left anterior oblique (LAO) view of the right coronary artery (RCA). **A:** Three-dimensional diagram of the 35-degree LAO view. **B:** Angiogram of the 35-degree LAO view. The posterior descending artery branch in this view is typically the most inferior vessel arising from the distal RCA. In cases of severe obstructions of the left anterior descending artery (LAD), it is important to maintain cine long enough to visualize collaterals from the distal RCA or from the conus branch to the LAD.

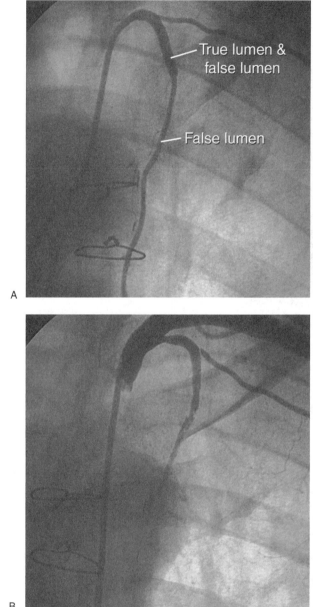

FIG. 3-7. Iatrogenic dissection of a left internal mammary graft. **A:** Dissection of left internal mammary graft showing both the true and false lumen. The thicker proximal segment represents the true lumen plus the false lumen, and the thinner distal segment represents the false dissecting lumen. **B:** Next run shows thrombosed graft with absence of blood flow.

TROUBLESHOOTING

Air Embolism

While performing coronary arteriography, extreme caution should be exercised to avoid inadvertently injecting air into the coronary arteries. If this should occur, patients may develop chest pain with or without ST-segment elevation on the ECG monitor, or ventricular fibrillation as a complication. Saline and intracoronary nitroglycerin is repeatedly injected into the coronary artery to clear the air emboli.

Coronary Dissection

Injection of contrast when the catheter is against the wall of the coronary artery (ventricularization of the pressure waveform) may result in coronary dissection. With a dissection, contrast is not cleared from the artery wall after termination of the injection (Figure 3-7). Prompt percutaneous repair or coronary bypass surgery should be considered.

CORONARY ANOMALIES

The various coronary anomalies in order of frequency, are:

- LAD and LCX arising from separate ostia (0.5%) (Figure 3-8)
- Origin of the LCX from the right sinus of Valsalva (0.5%) (Figure 3-9)
- Origin of the RCA from the ascending aorta above the right sinus of Valsalva (0.2%) (Figure 3-10)
- Origin of the RCA from the left sinus of Valsalva (0.1%) (Figure 3-11)
- AV fistula (0.1%) (Figure 3-12)
- Origin of the LMT from the right sinus of Valsalva (0.02%) (Figure 3-13)

MYOCARDIAL BRIDGING

In myocardial bridging, portions of epicardial coronary arteries (most commonly the LAD and the diagonals) run within the myocardium (Figure 3-14). Obliteration of the coronary lumen during systole with resolution in diastole may be seen. Because the majority of myocardial blood flow occurs in diastole, most cases of bridging are clinically benign as (98% 11-year survival). However, in rare situations, myocardial bridges may be associated with angina, myocardial ische-

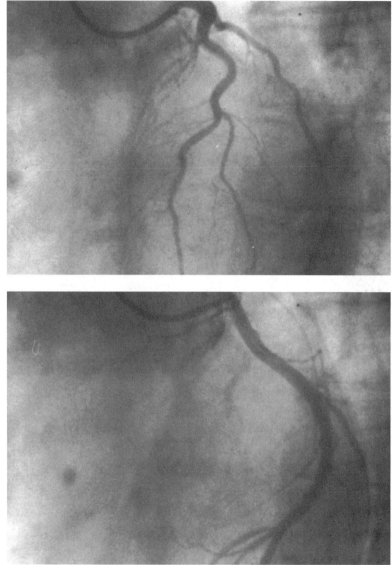

FIG. 3-8. Left anterior descending and left circumflex arteries arise from separate orifices. Panels **A** and **B** show selective engagement of the left anterior descending and the left circumflex arteries.

mia, myocardial infarction, left ventricular dysfunction, myocardial stunning, paroxysmal AV blockade, exercise-induced ventricular tachycardia, or sudden cardiac death. Effective therapies include beta-blockade and, in severe cases, coronary stenting or surgical myotomy with or without concomitant bypass surgery.

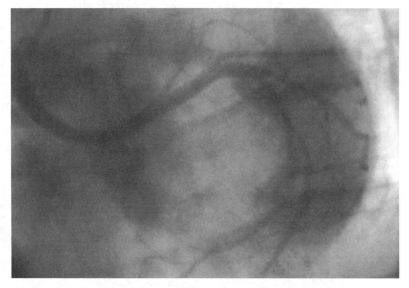

FIG. 3-9. Left circumflex artery arising from the right sinus of Valsalva. Left anterior oblique (LAO) projection of anomalous circumflex from right sinus of Valsalva passes inferior and posterior to aorta where it reaches the left atrioventricular groove and distributes normally over the lateral wall of the heart. In the LAO projection, this anomaly has the appearance of the letter "S" or "question mark" on its side.

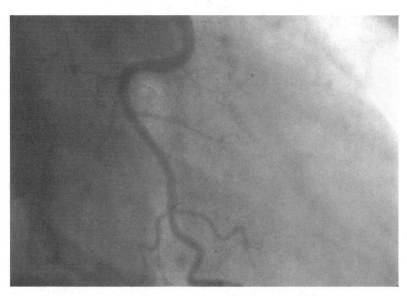

FIG. 3-10. Right coronary artery (RCA) arising from the ascending aorta above the right sinus of Valsalva. RCA arises from the ascending aorta above the right sinus of Valsalva, right anterior oblique projection. Note that the initial segment of this vessel is vertically oriented.

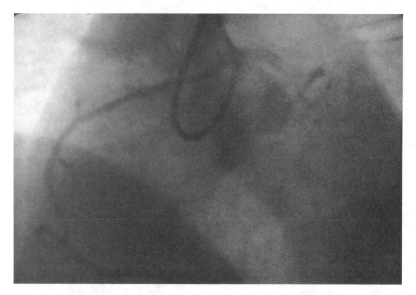

FIG. 3-11. Right coronary artery (RCA) arising from the left sinus of Valsalva. Anomalous RCA arises from the left sinus of Valsalva passing between the aorta and the pulmonary artery and to the right atrioventricular groove before distributing normally, left anterior oblique projection. Patients with this anomaly are at increased risk for sudden death, and it requires surgical correction.

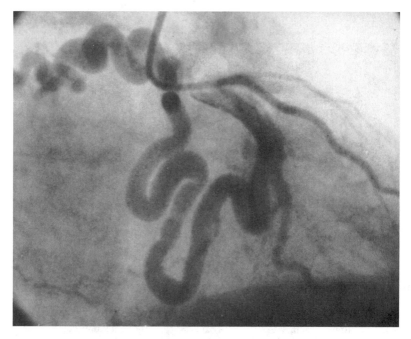

FIG. 3-12. Atrioventricular (AV) fistula arising from left circumflex artery (LCX) draining into superior vena cava. Serpiginous course of an AV fistula arising from LCX and draining into the superior vena cava, right anterior oblique projection.

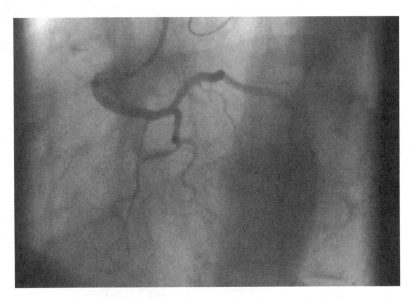

FIG. 3-13. Left main trunk (LMT) arising from the right sinus of Valsalva. Anomalous origin of the LMT from the right sinus of Valsalva. Selective visualization of the left coronary artery, left anterior oblique projection. The LMT arises from the right sinus of Valsalva and passes into the interventricular septum where is gives off a septal perforator. The vessel then reaches the epicardial surface of the heart where it divides into the left anterior descending and left circumflex arteries, which distribute normally.

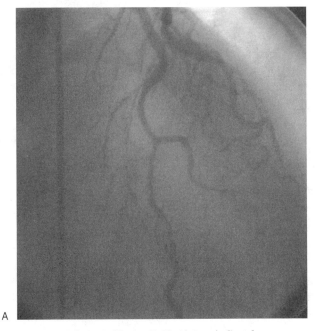

A

FIG. 3-14. Myocardial bridging. **A:** Systole.

(continued)

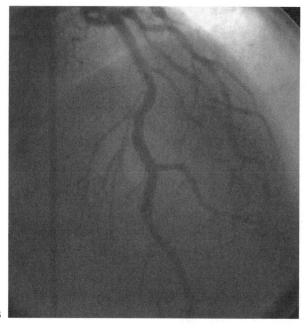

B

FIG. 3-14. *(Continued).* **B:** Diastole. Hypertrophied myocardium is seen compressing the midportion of the left anterior descending artery during systole.

SUGGESTED READINGS

Bashore TM, et al. American College of Cardiology/Society for Cardiac Angiography and Interventions clinical expert consensus document on cardiac catheterization laboratory standards. *J Am Coll Cardiol* 2001;37: 2170–2214.

Baum S. *Abram's angiography*, 4th ed. Boston: Little, Brown and Company, 1997:241–252.

Ellis SG. Role of coronary angiography. In: Fuster V, Ross R, Topol EJ, eds. *Atherosclerosis and coronary artery disease*, Vol. 2. Philadelphia: Lippincott–Raven Publishers, 1996:1433–1450.

Green CE. *Coronary cinematography*. Philadelphia: Lippincott–Raven Publishers, 1996:39–68.

Heupler FA, Proudfit WL, Razavi M, et al. Ergonovine maleate provocative test for coronary arterial spasm. *Am J Cardiol* 1978;41:631–640.

Manske CL, Sprafka JM, Strony JT, et al. Contrast nephropathy in azotemic diabetic patients undergoing coronary angiography. *Am J Med* 1990;89:615–620.

Matthai WH, Kussmal WG, Krol J, et al. A comparison of low- with high-osmolar contrast agents in cardiac angiography: identification of criteria for selective use. *Circulation* 1994;89:291–301.

Tilkian AG, Daily EK. *Cardiovascular procedures: diagnostic techniques and therapeutic procedures*. St. Louis: Mosby, 1986:117–151.

Yamanaka O, Hobbs RE. Coronary artery anomalies in 126,595 patients undergoing coronary arteriography. *Catheter Cardiovasc Diagn* 1990;21: 28–40.

4. BYPASS GRAFT ANGIOGRAPHY

J. Christopher Merritt and Frederick A. Heupler, Jr.

Saphenous Vein Grafts
Internal Mammary Artery Grafts
Radial Artery Grafts
Gastroepiploic Artery Grafts

Selective angiography of saphenous vein and arterial bypass grafts is usually performed immediately after angiography of the native coronary anatomy. The technique for bypass graft opacification is similar to that employed for native artery angiography. Knowledge of common graft locations and familiarity with multiple catheter types is essential for performing a complete study.

SAPHENOUS VEIN GRAFTS

Saphenous veins are the most commonly employed conduits in coronary revascularization. Approximately 87% of saphenous vein grafts (SVGs) remain patent at 6 months, with the patency rates dropping to approximately 63% at 10 years. Because of the high incidence of graft attrition, repeat revascularization often becomes necessary, requiring coronary angiography to assess graft patency.

The proximal anastomosis of most aortocoronary SVGs lies on the anterior surface of the aorta, several centimeters above the sinuses of Valsalva. Usually, the location of the various grafts in relation to one another follows a predictable sequence. Grafts to the left circumflex artery (LCX) are typically placed most superior, followed by grafts to the diagonal branches, LAD, and RCA (Figure 4-1). It should be noted, however, that because of variations in surgical technique, exceptions to this rule commonly exist. **If prior angiograms are available, they should be reviewed firsthand.**

The Judkins 4 French (F) right catheter (JR4) is the most common catheter employed in pursuit of vein grafts. **Typically, grafts to the right coronary artery (RCA) can be best visualized and cannulated while in the left anterior oblique (LAO) projection; grafts to the left coronary artery (LCA) system are most easily found while in the right anterior oblique (RAO) projection (Table 4-1).** The proximal anastomosis sites of these grafts lie superior to the native coronary ostia. Some surgeons place ostial

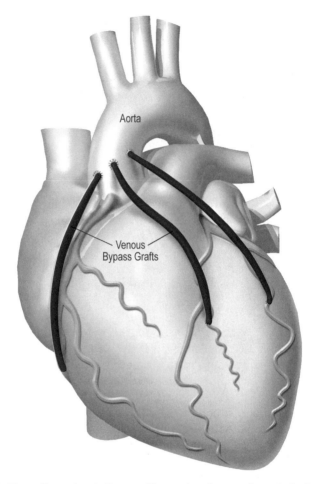

FIG. 4-1. Three-dimensional diagram illustrating the usual surgical placement of saphenous vein grafts. From superior to inferior in the aorta, the grafts anastomose to the lateral circumflex (OM), diagonal, and right coronary arteries.

TABLE 4-1. GENERAL GRAFT VIEWS

Graft	Ostium and Body	Distal Anastomosis	Native Artery
LIMA → LAD or SVG → LAD	Straight LAO and RAO	Left lateral view; LAO cranial	PA cranial
SVG → diagonal	Straight LAO and RAO	RAO cranial	LAO cranial
SVG→ LCX	Straight LAO and RAO	RAO caudal	RAO caudal
SVG → RCA	Straight LAO and RAO	LAO	PA cranial

LAD, left anterior descending; LAO, left anterior oblique; LCX, left circumflex coronary artery; LIMA, left internal mammary artery; PA, posteroanterior; RAO, right anterior oblique; SVG, saphenous vein graft.

graft markers on the outer surface of the aorta during surgery to facilitate location of the grafts for future catheterizations. Surgical clips may also provide clues as to the location of grafts.

Steady up-and-down movements of the catheter in the ascending aorta, typically from the second to the fourth sternal sutures, facilitate engagement of the various grafts. The catheter tip often "jumps" forward when it cannulates an ostium. Damping of the pressure waveform may indicate that the catheter tip is lying against the vessel wall, or that there is an ostial stenosis. In this situation, the catheter should be cautiously withdrawn while simultaneously reversing its torque. Occasionally, the pressure waveform remains damped and it may be necessary to perform a ramped injection of contrast with quick removal of the catheter to rule out critical stenoses or subtotal obstruction of a graft. Remember that a deep-seated catheter that lies beyond the ostium may fail to define a significant proximal stenosis. Occluded grafts will appear as a stump upon selective injection.

If a graft cannot be located, do not assume that the graft is occluded. Other catheters with different angulation may be necessary. **If further attempts fail, aortography may be helpful in locating difficult-to-find grafts.**

A careful review of native coronary artery arteriograms may also provide clues regarding graft patency. For instance, if a bypassed native artery demonstrates retrograde graft filling or competitive distal flow, the graft supplying that artery is likely patent. Conversely, if normal distal flow is seen in the bypassed native artery without competitive filling, the graft is probably occluded.

TROUBLESHOOTING
Cannulating "Difficult" Grafts

SVG to LCA: This graft is usually the most cranially located graft within the ascending aorta. It is best engaged with a JR4 catheter while in the RAO projection, as are all grafts to the LCA system. Gentle clockwise rotation of the catheter at a location in the ascending aorta above the other SVGs will often successfully find the graft ostium. With all LCA grafts, the operator should strive to position the tip of the catheter so that it faces toward the right side of the aortic silhouette in the RAO view. Once engaged, the usual LAO and RAO views are obtained.

SVG to left anterior descending artery (LAD) and diagonal branches: The LAD graft is most commonly located above the ostium of the native LCA, and just beneath the ostium of the LCX graft described above. Again, with the JR4 catheter lying in the ascending aorta, clockwise rotation of the catheter usually locates the ostium of this graft. It often helps to rotate the catheter slightly above the suspected location of the ostium, as clockwise rotation usually brings the tip downward slightly.

SVG to RCA: This graft is commonly placed just above the native RCA ostium. Simply withdrawing the JR4 catheter from the RCA will often cannulate the graft ostium. If this fails, clockwise rotation of the catheter a few centimeters above the native RCA may bring the catheter into the correct plane. Sometimes the takeoff of the RCA graft is at an acute angle from the aorta and is not easily cannulated with the JR4 catheter. A multipurpose catheter can be helpful in such circumstances. Gentle clockwise rotation as this catheter is first withdrawn, then advanced toward such a downwardly directed graft will usually place the catheter within the ostium. Right modified Amplatz, right coronary bypass, and 3DRC (Cordis Corp., Miami, FL, U.S.A.) catheters are other alternatives.

Once properly engaged, each graft should be visualized in both the left and RAO projections using an injection technique similar to that employed for native coronaries. Usually, several views are needed to fully assess the graft ostium, body, and distal anastomosis.

INTERNAL MAMMARY ARTERY GRAFTS

Internal mammary artery (IMA) grafts are used routinely in coronary artery bypass surgery, as they provide superior patency rates compared to venous grafts. Left internal mammary artery (LIMA) graft patency has been reported to be 93% at 6 months and 90% at 10 years. When these arterial grafts do fail, **the culprit stenosis usually lies at the distal anastomosis or in the artery just beyond the anastomosis.**

To successfully cannulate the LIMA, the operator must understand the anatomy of the left subclavian artery and its branches. The LIMA is often anastomosed to the mid- or distal LAD, although it is sometimes attached to diagonal branches or the LCX instead. It typically arises anteroinferiorly from the left subclavian artery, 1 to 3 cm beyond the vertebral artery (Figure 4-2).

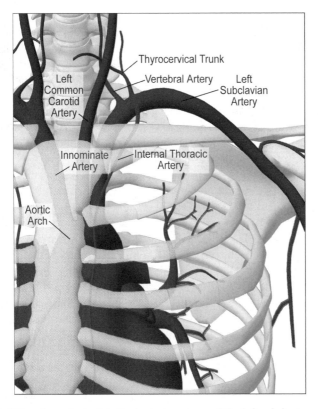

FIG. 4-2. This schematic depicts the typical anatomy of the left subclavian artery and its most proximal branches. Note that the internal mammary (thoracic) artery arises anteroinferiorly. Remember that when evaluating a patient with ischemia in the internal mammary artery (IMA) distribution, it is important to rule out the possibility of subclavian or innominate stenosis proximal to the IMA origin.

Using the LAO projection, the JR4 catheter is positioned in the aortic arch just proximal to the origin of the left subclavian artery. The catheter is then slowly pulled back as gentle counterclockwise rotation is applied, thereby moving the tip of the catheter into the origin of the left subclavian artery. An alternative technique for subclavian artery cannulation involves extending the tip of the JR4 catheter just past the left subclavian origin, then rotating the catheter clockwise to engage the artery. An angiogram of this artery in the PA projection enables the operator to locate the ostium of the LIMA and exclude a significant subclavian stenosis that could be indirectly causing myocardial ischemia. When the subclavian artery is tortuous, the origin of the LIMA is often better demonstrated in the RAO projection.

A guidewire [either the J-tip or Wholey (Mallinckrodt, Hazelwood, MO, U.S.A.)] is then advanced gently through the catheter into the subclavian artery and out into the axillary artery, well beyond the origin of the LIMA. At this point, the catheter should be advanced over the guidewire to a point about halfway between the sternum and the left shoulder. The guidewire is then removed and the catheter flushed vigorously. To engage the LIMA, the catheter is slowly withdrawn while simultaneously applying gentle counter-clockwise rotation so that the catheter tip faces anteriorly. Because the LIMA often arises from the subclavian artery at a 90-degree angle, a catheter with a sharper curve, such as the LIMA or Special 5F IMA catheter, may be necessary.

Small test injections can be used to orient the operator. **Nonionic contrast is advisable when injecting the subclavian and internal mammary arteries** in order to minimize the risk of hyperosmolar neurotoxicity, as well as reduce the burning discomfort to the patient. Having the patient turn his/her head to the left or right can help engage the graft by slightly changing the orientation of the catheter.

Once the catheter cannulates the mammary graft, the tip may "jump" into the ostium. One has to be very cautious when manipulating the catheter near or within the LIMA, as this vessel is especially delicate and prone to dissection (see Figure 3-7). For this reason, fine movements are advisable whenever attempting to engage the LIMA. If pressure damping does occur, the catheter tip should quickly and carefully be rotated out of the artery.

Once engaged, the LIMA graft is injected in at least two projections, paying special attention to the anastomotic site. Forceful injections are discouraged. Straight RAO and LAO projections are most commonly employed. Cranial angulation can be added to either projection to better visualize the distal aspect of the LAD. A cross-table lateral view is sometimes helpful to gain an additional view of the anastomotic site.

If the LIMA cannot be selectively engaged, a subselective view can be obtained. In this instance, the catheter should be positioned as close as possible to the LIMA ostium. A blood pressure cuff inflated on the left arm will help direct contrast flow preferentially down the LIMA instead of distally into the brachial artery.

Selective visualization of the right internal mammary artery (RIMA) is similar to that of the LIMA above, but it is more difficult. A JR4 or LIMA catheter (there is no specific RIMA catheter) is advanced into the proximal aortic arch past the origin of the innominate artery. Counterclockwise rotation will bring the tip of the catheter into this artery's origin. Again, a guidewire is advanced through the catheter down the right subclavian artery, taking great care to avoid the right common carotid artery. The catheter is then advanced over the guidewire just as in LIMA catheterization. The difference here is that upon pulling back the catheter, slow clockwise rotation is applied to bring the tip anteriorly to engage the RIMA ostium. When it is impossible to cannulate the RIMA with this technique, the operator may elect to configure a JR4 or LIMA catheter with a concave secondary curve proximal to the primary curve.

The RIMA is often used as a "free" graft, with its proximal anastomosis in the ascending aorta. In this case, the procedure for cannulating the graft is the same as that for saphenous vein grafts.

RADIAL ARTERY GRAFTS

On occasion, the operator may encounter a radial artery graft. Emerging data suggests that short-term patency of radial artery grafts is comparable to that of SVGs. Further data regarding long-term patency are not available. Radial artery grafts are often placed in similar locations as SVGs, and they are cannulated in much the same way. Angiographically, these grafts have a smaller caliber and smoother appearance than their SVG counterparts.

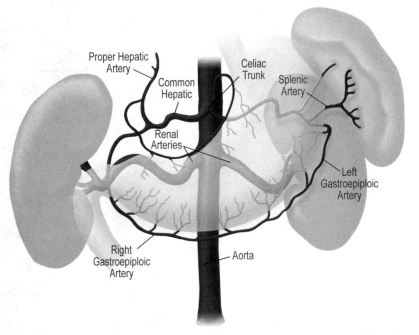

FIG. 4-3. Schematic diagram depicting normal abdominal aorta anatomy. Note that the gastroepiploic artery is a branch of the common hepatic artery, which originates from the celiac trunk. The celiac trunk is typically located along the anterior aorta just proximal to the 12th thoracic vertebra.

GASTROEPIPLOIC ARTERY GRAFTS

The gastroepiploic artery (Figure 4-3) is a branch of the gastroduodenal artery, which originates from the common hepatic artery of the celiac trunk. It usually serves as an *in situ* graft to a vessel along the inferior surface of the heart, such as the PDA. The graft is usually catheterized with the use of a standard visceral catheter, such as the Cobra (Terumo, Frankfurt/Main, Germany) catheter. Subselective artery cannulation may erroneously lead to the conclusion that the graft is occluded, so it is important to selectively engage the artery.

SUGGESTED READINGS

Hamm CW, Reimers J, Ischinger T, et al. A randomized study of coronary angioplasty compared with bypass surgery in patients with symptomatic multivessel coronary disease. German Angioplasty Bypass Surgery Investigation (GABI) *N Engl J Med* 1994;331:1037–1043.

Isshiki T, Yamaguchi T, Nakamura T, et al. Postoperative angiographic evaluation of gastroepiploic artery grafts. *Cathet Cardiovasc Diagn* 1990;21: 233–238.

Lytle BW, Cosgrove DM 3rd. Coronary artery bypass surgery. *Curr Probl Surg* 992;29:733–807.

Peterson KL, Nicod P. *Cardiac catheterization: methods, diagnosis, and therapy*. Philadelphia: WB Saunders Co., 1997.

Tatoulis J, Royse AG, Buxton BF, et al. The radial artery in coronary surgery: a 5-year experience—clinical and angiographic results. *Ann Thoracic Surg* 2002;73:143–147.

Tixier DB, Acar C, Carpentier AF. Coronary-coronary Bypass using the radial artery. *Ann Thorac Surg* 1995;60:693.

5. LEFT VENTIRICULOGRAPHY AND AORTOGRAPHY

Deepak Vivekananthan and Frederick A. Heupler, Jr.

Left Ventriculography
  Preparation
  Entering the Ventricle
  Views
  Analysis
  Complications
Aortography
  Preparation
  Views
  Analysis

LEFT VENTRICULOGRAPHY

Left ventriculography provides important anatomic and functional information that supplements coronary angiography (Table 5-1). Single-plane ventriculography is routinely performed in most catheterization laboratories, but some operators prefer biplane ventriculography because it provides more detailed information about ventricular anatomy and function. Biplane ventriculography does have limitations, such as costly angiographic equipment, additional radiation exposure to both operator and patient, and longer angiographic setup time. When a patient is unstable hemodynamically, it is usually advisable to forego ventriculography. Additional contraindications are listed in Table 5-2.

Preparation

The Medrad (Indianola, PA, U.S.A.) powered flow injector is connected to extension tubing and loaded with contrast. During this process, air bubbles should be purged from the injector. Once appropriate pressure measurements have been obtained, the pigtail catheter is connected to the extension tubing from the power injec-

TABLE 5-1. INDICATIONS FOR LEFT VENTRICULOGRAPHY

Assessment of global left ventricular systolic function and regional wall motion
Assessment of severity of mitral regurgitation
Identification and assessment of muscular and membranous ventricular septal defects

TABLE 5-2. CONTRAINDICATIONS FOR LEFT VENTRICULOGRAPHY

Critical left main disease
Critical aortic stenosis
Fresh intracardiac thrombus[a]
Tilting-disc aortic prosthesis
Decompensated heart failure and/or renal failure

[a]Because sessile thrombi >6 mo old have a lower risk of dislodgement, some operators will proceed with ventriculography in this circumstance.

tor via a blood-contrast interface to minimize the risk of air embolism with left ventriculography. Usually the left ventricular cavity is adequately visualized with 30 to 50 mL of contrast.

The parameters listed in Table 5-3 can serve as a baseline when deciding on the rate and volume of contrast injection. Of course, certain patient characteristics and clinical settings will influence these settings. For instance, in patients with known or suspected severe mitral regurgitation, at least 50 to 60 mL of contrast dye is usually needed to completely opacify the left atrium. Higher rates of contrast injection are also needed in patients with high cardiac outputs and/or dilatated left ventricular cavities. Conversely, patients with smaller ventricular cavities, such as elderly females, or those with hypertensive heart disease, may need only 30 to 36 mL of contrast dye to provide adequate imaging. **All patients with hemodynamically significant valvular disease, left ventricular dysfunction, or elevated left-ventricular end-diastolic pressure should receive nonionic contrast for ventriculography**

Entering the Ventricle

The catheter most commonly used for ventriculography is a 6 French (F) angled pigtail catheter. The distal segment of this catheter should be angled 145 to 155 degrees to facilitate passage into the left ventricle while simultaneously preventing the endhole from contacting the endocardium, reducing the risk of endocardial staining. The multiple side-holes help dissipate the pressure of rapid power contrast injection, thereby preventing excessive catheter movement.

TABLE 5-3. STANDARD SETTINGS FOR LEFT VENTRICULOGRAPHY

Rate of rise	0–0.4 sec
Rate of injection	10–15 mL/sec
Volume of injection	30–40 mL
Maximum pressure	600–700 psi

psi, pounds per square inch.

The pigtail catheter is advanced over a 0.035-in. J-tip guidewire to a position in the ascending aorta just superior to the aortic valve. The tip should be pointed towards the orifice of the valve and the catheter rotated so that the pigtail loop resembles a "6". In this position, gently advancing the catheter will usually push it across the valve orifice and into the ventricle.

Occasionally, the pigtail catheter will prolapse into the ventricle while the pigtail remains in the ascending aorta. Slowly advancing the guidewire through the terminal portion of the catheter should provide enough additional support to allow entry into the ventricle. Once in the ventricle, the tip of the pigtail should be positioned in the center of the cavity (Figure 5-1).

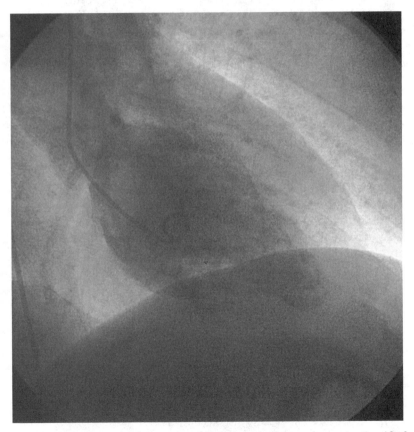

FIG. 5-1. Thirty-degree right anterior oblique ventriculogram demonstrating ideal placement of the pigtail catheter in the ventricular mid-cavity. The most common reasons for ectopy during ventriculography are contact of the catheter with either the apex or the septum. Gentle counterclockwise rotation and/or pullback of the catheter should eliminate the ectopy.

TROUBLESHOOTING
Ventricular Ectopy

If the pigtail catheter irritates the apex, the risk of ventricular ectopy rises significantly. Gentle counterclockwise rotation and pullback should separate the catheter from the septal and apical walls, and the ectopy will usually resolve.

Entrapment in Mitral Valve Apparatus

Occasionally the catheter tip may become trapped within the mitral valve apparatus. If ventriculography is performed under these circumstances, transient but significant mitral regurgitation may develop. Gentle clockwise rotation should dislodge the catheter from the apparatus and place it in the center of the ventricle. If not, the catheter can be withdrawn from the ventricle and ventricular entry reattempted.

Once the catheter is stabilized within the left ventricle, it is connected to the pressure manifold, flushed, and used to record intraventricular pressures. Systolic pressure is typically recorded on a 200-mm Hg scale, while left ventricular end-diastolic pressure (LVEDP) is best appreciated on a 40-mm Hg scale. **Markedly elevated LVEDP (greater than 30mm Hg) usually precludes left ventriculography.** Sometimes the administration of sublingual nitroglycerin will reduce LVEDP to a more acceptable level.

In a patient with compromised left ventricular systolic function and/or markedly elevated LVEDP, a hand-injection left ventriculogram using digital subtraction angiography may be preferred. In this circumstance, usually no more than 10 mL of contrast is needed.

TROUBLESHOOTING
Crossing a Stenotic Aortic Valve

As a general rule, it should be understood that crossing a stenotic aortic valve requires patience, experience, and a bit of luck. This task can be accomplished with a variety of catheters and wires depending on operator preference, experience and patient anatomy. Some operators prefer a brief cine run of aortic valve opening and closing in right anterior oblique (RAO) and left anterior oblique (LAO) projections to identify the angle and plane of the aortic valve orifice prior to crossing it.

Usually the aortic valve can be crossed with an angled pigtail catheter using the previously described approach. However, in cases of severe aortic stenosis, alternative techniques may be preferred. Because of the inherent thrombogenicity of guidewires, some operators advise administering 5,000 U of unfractionated heparin before attempting to cross a stenotic aortic valve. In addition, after every 3 minutes of unsuccessful wire manipulation, the wire should be removed and wiped, and the catheter should be flushed vigorously to prevent thrombus formation. Under no circumstance, should excessive force ever be used to pass the wire into the left ventricle. The most common techniques are reviewed below.

Wire Selection

The most common wires utilized to cross a severely stenotic aortic valve are a straight-tip (0.035 or 0.038) or Rosen exchange J-tip (Cook Inc., Bloomington, IN, U.S.A.) The Rosen wire is a J-tip wire with a J-curve that is narrower (5-mm diameter) than the usual J-tip (10-mm diameter). The advantage of the Rosen wire is that the J-tip eliminates the risk of left ventricular perforation, but it may be more difficult to pass across a very severely stenotic valve. The advantage of a straight-tip wire is that it will cross virtually any stenotic aortic valve, but the straight tip can perforate the left ventricle. The safest procedure is to initially attempt to cross the valve with the Rosen wire, which can be accomplished in more than 90% of cases.

Catheter Selection

Common catheters utilized to cross the aortic valve are the pigtail, Amplatz left coronary, Feldman, Judkins right coronary, and multipurpose catheters. The Amplatz and Feldman catheters are preferred if the aorta is dilatated. The length of the secondary curve of these catheters should be adjusted proportionally to the diameter of the aorta. The Judkins right coronary and multipurpose catheters are preferred when the aortic root is narrow.

Technique

Once the selected catheter is positioned in the ascending aorta, the guidewire is cautiously advanced through the endhole of the catheter in an attempt to cross the valve orifice. Carefully advancing and rotating the catheter simultaneously should eventually direct the wire across the aortic valve. The tip of the wire should be directed anteriorly and to the patient's left. Generally, it is easier to cross the valve in the RAO projection. The operator should attempt to advance the wire across the valve during systole. Altering the amount of wire protruding from the pigtail catheter may help direct the wire. For instance, more wire protruding from the pigtail catheter directs the wire towards the right coronary sinus, whereas less wire protruding directs the wire to the left coronary sinus.

Crossing a Prosthetic Aortic Valve

From a clinical standpoint, crossing a stenotic aortic valve to measure the gradient is most important in the following circumstances: when echocardiography provides suboptimal image quality, when echocardiographic and clinical findings do not correlate, and when there is severe left ventricular dysfunction with low cardiac output. It is absolutely contraindicated to cross a tilting-disc aortic valve prosthesis [St. Jude (St. Jude Medical, St. Paul, MN, U.S.A.), Medtronic-Hall (Medtronic, Inc., Minneapolis, MN, U.S.A.), Bjork–Shiley]. Attempts at catheter or wire passage across these prostheses could result in entrapment and/or disc dislodgement. Bioprosthetic porcine and pericardial valves may be crossed. In theory, Starr-Edwards (Edwards Lifesciences, Irvine, CA, U.S.A.) prosthetic valves may also be crossed, but smaller sized catheters are usually necessary. Avoid crossing a metal prosthesis unless absolutely necessary.

Views

The most common views for left ventriculography are the 30-degree RAO and 60-degree LAO views. The optimal magnification is usually a 9-in. field, because it allows for complete visualization of the entire left ventricle, including both the mitral and aortic valves, without panning.

30-Degree Right Anterior Oblique View

The 30-degree RAO view is particularly helpful because it projects the left ventricle off the spine, thus producing a higher-quality picture (Figure 5-2). Positioning the wedge filter into the upper right hand corner usually improves image quality. The walls best visual-

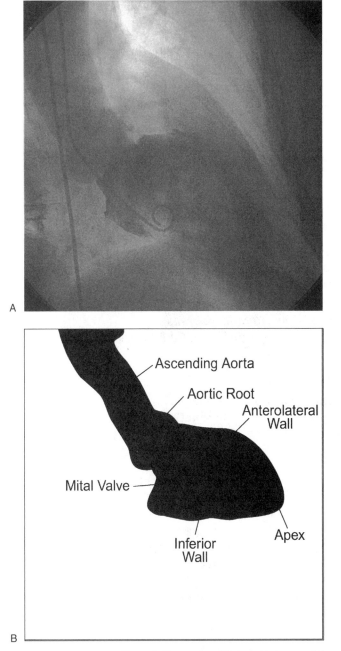

FIG. 5-2. Left ventriculogram **(A)** and illustration **(B)** in a 30-degree right anterior oblique view.

ized with the 30-degree RAO view include the anterior, apical, and inferior walls. Also, from this angle the mitral valve is seen in profile, allowing for evaluation of mitral valve disease. One limitation of this view is that it places the left atrium over the spine and descending aorta, thus impairing the operator's ability to evaluate the severity of mitral regurgitation. Adding steeper RAO angulation (45 degrees) will help the operator quantify mitral regurgitation since this view positions the left atrium to the right of the spine.

60-Degree Left Anterior Oblique View

The 60-degree LAO view is most useful for functional assessment of the ventricular septum, lateral wall, and posterior walls (Figure 5-3). Also, the aortic valve is well visualized. Adding 25 degrees of cranial angulation reduces any foreshortening of the ventricular septum and therefore is ideal - for assessing the left ventricular outflow tract and a muscular ventricular septal defect. Cranial angulation also provides improved visualization of the left atrium because it positions the left atrium away from the spine, the left ventricle, and the descending aorta.

Left lateral view (70 to 80 degrees)

A lateral view is especially helpful for assessment of a membranous ventricular septal defect.

Analysis

Left Ventricular Systolic Function

In most laboratories, a qualitative assessment of left ventricular systolic function, mitral regurgitation severity, and regional wall motion is performed. When describing regional wall motion, the walls are commonly classified as either normal, hypokinetic, akinetic, or dyskinetic (Table 5-4). Once all the ventricular walls have been studied, an estimation of global left ventricular systolic function is made. Usually, this estimation is done semiquantitatively (Table 5-5). A quantitative assessment of left ventricular systolic function is calculated in some laboratories by comparing end-systolic to end-diastolic left ventricular volume. However, these calculations are rarely done on a routine basis.

Valvular Anatomy and Function

During left ventriculography, both aortic and mitral valve function should be grossly assessed. Table 5-6 classifies degrees of mitral regurgitation. Leaflet mobility, thickening, and calcification can each be evaluated. Mitral annular calcification, if present, should be noted and quantified. Bicuspid aortic valves and mitral valve prolapse might also be observed, and deserve mention and description.

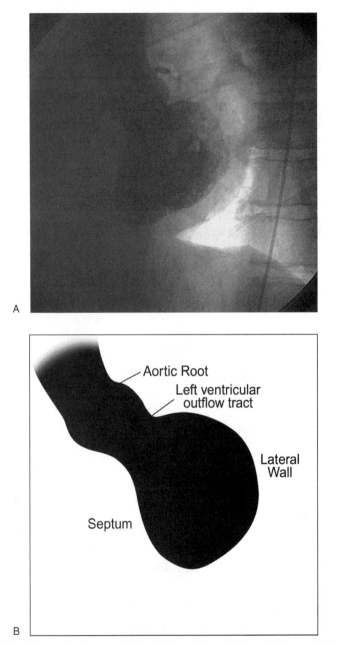

FIG. 5-3. Left ventriculogram **(A)** and illustration **(B)** in a 60-degree left anterior oblique view.

TABLE 5-4. **CLASSIFICATION OF REGIONAL WALL MOTION**

Hypokinesia	Reduction of inward motion during systole
Akinesia	Absence of inward motion during systole
Dyskinesia	Paradoxical outward motion during systole

Prosthetic Valves

The ideal angulation for either the RAO or LAO view will place the annulus of the prosthesis perpendicular to the imaging plane. **The best angle for evaluating mitral valve function is an RAO view (Figure 5-4).** The best angle for evaluating aortic valve function is an LAO view (Figure 5-5) .

A complete fluoroscopic evaluation includes assessment of valvular motion and structural integrity. Some prosthetic valve companies, such as St. Jude's and Bjork–Shiley, publish what they consider to be normal parameters for opening and closing angles. These angles can be measured fluoroscopically to determine if a specific valve is functioning properly. As a general rule, however, the availability of multiplane transesophageal echocardiography (TEE) obviates the need for angiographic assessment of prosthetic valve function in most cases.

Complications

The complications of left ventriculography are listed in Table 5-7.

AORTOGRAPHY

Aortography is not routinely performed during diagnostic cardiac catheterization. However, in certain circumstances (Table 5-8), it may be necessary to better define aortic root anatomy and aortic valvular function (Table 5-9). Contraindications to aortography are listed in Table 5-10.

Preparation

A 6F pigtail catheter is most commonly employed because its multiple side-holes reduce the risk for aortic dissection during power injection. Ideally, the pigtail is advanced to a location just above the

TABLE 5-5. **SEMIQUANTITATIVE ASSESSMENT OF LEFT VENTRICULAR SYSTOLIC FUNCTION**

Left Ventricular Systolic Function	Ejection Fraction
Normal	≥ 55%–60%
Low normal	50%
Mildly impaired	40%–49%
Moderately impaired	30%–39%
Severely impaired	≤ 30%

TABLE 5-6. ANGIOGRAPHIC ASSESSMENT OF MITRAL REGURGITATION

Grade	Angiographic Appearance
Mild (1+)	Faint LA opacification that clears with each beat Does not opacify the entire LA
Moderate (2+)	Complete LA opacification after several beats Opacification intensity: LA<LV
Moderately severe (3+)	Complete LA opacification Opacification intensity: LA=LV
Severe (4+)	Complete LA opacification after one beat Opacification intensity: LA>LV Opacification of pulmonary veins

LA, left atrium/atrial; LV, left ventricle.

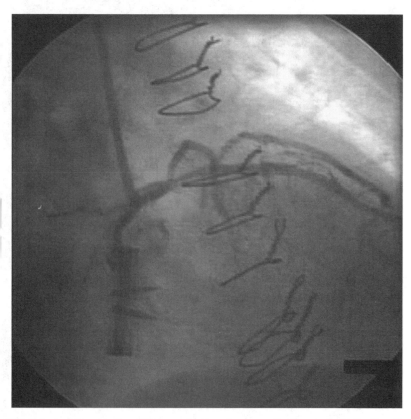

FIG. 5-4. A right anterior oblique projection of a normally functioning bileaflet tilting disc (St. Jude's) mitral valve prosthesis. (Courtesy of Mario Garcia, M.D., Cleveland Foundation Clinic, Cleveland, OH, U.S.A.)

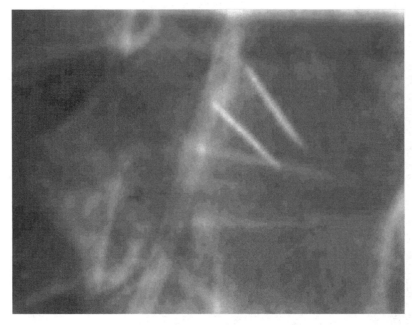

FIG. 5-5. A left anterior oblique projection of a normally functioning bileaflet tilting disc aortic valve prosthesis. (Courtesy of Mario Garcia, M.D.)

TABLE 5-7. **COMPLICATIONS OF LEFT VENTRICULOGRAPHY**

Complication	Caveats
Ventricular arrhythmias	Most common complication Sustained VT is an indication for immediate wire/catheter removal
Complete heart block	Complete heart block may occur due to trauma from the catheter as it enters the left ventricle or during ventriculography. Particular caution should be used in patients with baseline RBBB and left posterior hemiblock
Endocardial staining	Refers to accumulation of contrast within endocardium Larger stains may result in VT or VFl
Air embolism	Potentially catastrophic complication, which may result in CVA or MI
Cardiac tamponade	Catastrophic complication that occurs when ventricle is punctured during aggressive wire manipulation (occurred in about 0.3% of patients in one series)

CVA, cerebrovascular accident; LVOT, left ventricular outflow tract; MI, myocardial infarction; RBBB, right bundle branch block; VFl, ventricular flutter; VT, ventricular tachycardia.

TABLE 5-8. COMMON INDICATIONS FOR AORTOGRAPHY

Assess severity of aortic regurgitation
Assess aneurysm size
Identify the location and extent of aortic dissection
Locate/opacify bypass grafts or anomalous coronary arteries
Localize coarctation of the aorta

sinotubular junction. Standard injection volume and rate is 40 to 60 mL at 20 mL/sec.

Views

The most useful view is a 60-degree LAO view because both the aortic root anatomy and the severity of aortic insufficiency can be evaluated (Figure 5-6 and Table 5-11).

Analysis

To measure aortic root size, image acquisition of a standard-sized object, often a radiopaque ball, is used as a reference (Figure 5-7). The diameter of this object is measured during angiography and then used to calculate the diameter of the aortic root. Once an image of the object has been obtained, aortic root angiography must be performed with the same magnification and camera angle.

Assessment of Aortic Dissection

Aortography may help identify the origin and proximal and/or distal extension of an aortic dissection (Figure 5-8). In addition, the severity of aortic regurgitation, the patency of the proximal coronary arteries, and location of an intimal flap may also be evaluated. **With refinement of less invasive imaging modalities such as TEE, computed tomography scan, and cardiac magnetic resonance imaging, aortography is no longer the initial imaging modality of choice in the diagnosis of aortic dissection.**

TABLE 5-9. NORMAL AORTIC ANATOMY

Location	Description
Aortic root or bulb	Formed by the three sinuses of Valsalva (right, left, and posterior)
Ascending aorta	Measures 2.2–3.8 cm in diameter in normal adults
Aortic arch	Gives rise to the great vessels, including the brachiocephalic, left common carotid, and left subclavian artery
Descending aorta	Continuation of aorta distal to left subclavian artery
	Typically measures ~2.5 cm in diameter
	Anatomic landmark often used to distinguish type A from type B dissections

TABLE 5-10. CONTRAINDICATIONS TO AORTOGRAPHY

Severe heart failure
Renal failure

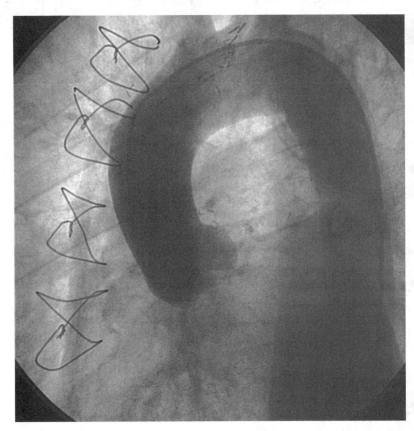

FIG. 5-6. Sixty-degree left anterior oblique aortography demonstrating a normal aorta.

TABLE 5-11. ANGIOGRAPHIC ASSESSMENT OF AORTIC INSUFFICIENCY

Grade	Angiographic Appearance
Mild (1+)	Faint, incomplete LV opacification that clears with each beat
Moderate (2+)	Opacification of LV < aorta
Moderately severe (3+)	Progressive opacification of entire LV=aorta
Severe (4+)	Dense LV opacification after one beat > aorta

LV, left ventricle/ventricular.

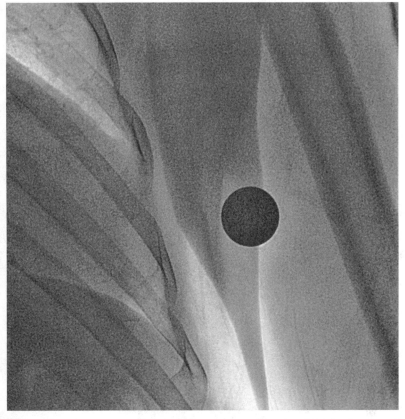

FIG. 5-7. An object with a predefined diameter may be placed in the fluoroscopic field, and used as a reference when measuring aortic aneurysms, for instance.

Locating Bypass Grafts

Aortography is sometimes used to help locate difficult-to-find bypass grafts. It is important to remember, however, that even if a bypass graft is not opacified by aortography, it does not completely rule out the presence of patent grafts.

Coarctation of the Aorta

Aortic coarctation is best appreciated with a lateral view (Figure 5-9). Aortography identifies the site of obstruction and extent of pre- and/or poststenotic dilatation. A pressure gradient greater than 20 mm Hg across the coarctation is considered to be hemodynamically significant, while a gradient greater than 50 mm Hg mandates intervention.

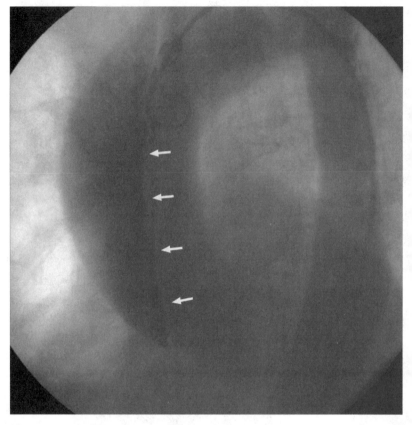

FIG. 5-8. An example of an ascending aortic dissection in left anterior oblique projection. Note the "flap" visualized (*arrows*).

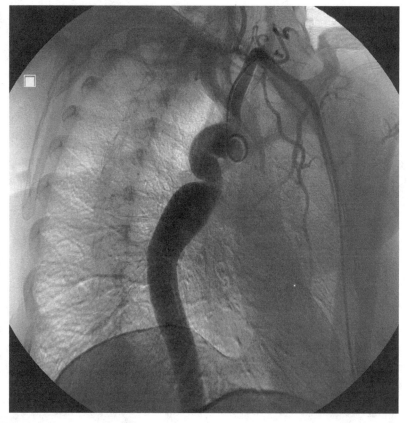

FIG. 5-9. Example of coarctation of the aorta in steep right anterior oblique projection.

SUGGESTED READINGS

Arciniegas JG, Soto B, Little WC, et al. Cineangiographs in the diagnosis of aortic dissection. *Am J Cardiol* 1981;47:890–894.

Bhargava V, Warren S, Vieweg WVR, et al. Quantitation of left ventricular wall motion in normal subjects: comparison of various methods. *Cathet Cardiovasc Diagn* 1980;6:7–16.

Chaitman BR, DeMots H, Bristow JD, et al. Objective and subjective analysis of left ventricular angiograms. *Circulation* 1975;52:420–425.

Feldman T, Carroll JD, Chiu YC. An improved catheter design for assessing stenosed aortic valves. *Cathet Cardiovasc Diagn* 1989;16:279–283.

6. HEMODYNAMICS IN THE CATH LAB

David Lee, Wilson H. Tang, and Frederick A. Heupler, Jr.

Hemodynamic data are an important part of every diagnostic catheterization, particularly in patients with cardiomyopathies, valvular disorders, and pericardial disease. The measurement of hemodynamics utilizes pressure, oximetry, and temperature differences to derive functional information about the heart. To fully understand hemodynamics, one must first learn how to make proper measurements, calculate derived values, and interpret the results in relation to specific disease conditions.

METHODOLOGY OF HEMODYNAMIC MEASUREMENTS

Pressure Measurements

The most accurate method for measuring pressures in the heart is to utilize a system with the pressure transducer (usually a strain-gauge type) located at the exact location of interest. However, while catheters with a pressure transducer at the tip are available, they are too expensive to be used routinely and are generally used for research purposes only. Thus, the most common method of measuring pressure in the cardiac catheterization lab utilizes a system incorporating a fluid-filled catheter connected through a manifold to a pressure transducer. This system, however, has several characteristics that influence its fidelity and accuracy. Because the pressure

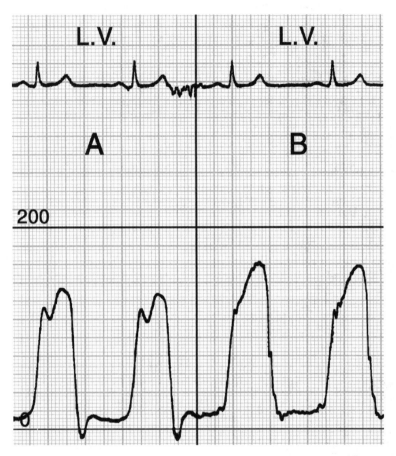

FIG. 6-1. Pressure underdamping caused by an air bubble in the tubing. This produces high-frequency oscillations that result in falsely elevated peak systolic pressures **(B)**. Corrected waveform **(A)**. *L.V.*, left ventricular pressure.

waveform is transmitted through fluid until it reaches the transducer outside the body, there is both a time delay and a damping of the pressure signal that usually filters out the high-frequency components. Underdamping of the system can be a problem, especially if air bubbles are present in the system (Figure 6-1). Other common sources of error are listed in Table 6-1.

TROUBLESHOOTING
Inserting Pulmonary Artery Catheter
1. Obtain vascular accesses, typically with an 8 French (F) catheter sheath, allowing passage of the 7F **pulmonary artery**

TABLE 6-1. **COMMON SOURCES OF ERROR IN HEMODYNAMIC MEASUREMENTS**

Source of Error	Result of Error	Correct Technique
Transducer position	Too-low pressure recorded if positioned too high	At level of mid-right atrium, halfway up the body between spine and sternum
Catheter bore	—	Maximize catheter bore size
Catheter length	—	Minimize length of tubing
Kink in tubing	—	Replace tubing or catheter
Fluid viscosity	Contrast in tubing	Catheter should be filled with normal saline; avoid contrast
Air in system	Air bubbles at connection points or transducer	Flush catheters and manifold to avoid presence of air bubbles
Tip positioning	"Catheter whip"	Reposition catheter
Stable arrhythmias	—	Average measurements over several beats to obtain an average

(PA) catheter. Typically, if the PA catheter is guided solely by pressure tracings to advance it to wedge position, the right internal jugular and left subclavian veins provide the most direct anatomic routes to the pulmonary artery that matches the natural curve of the catheter.

2. Inflate the balloon at the tip of the catheter under water to ensure there is no air leakage.
3. Make sure all lumens of the PA catheter are flushed.
4. Zero the pressure transducer at the level of the mid-right atrium.
5. Connect the PA catheter's distal (PA) port to the pressure transducer. Make sure there are no air bubbles in the tubing or catheter.
6. Advance the catheter 20 cm through the sheath prior to balloon inflation to ensure the catheter tip clears the sheath. Do not advance if any resistance is met.
7. Beware of arrhythmias, primarily premature ventricular contractions (PVCs) and nonsustained ventricular tachycardia, especially after the catheter crosses the tricuspid valve. In the setting of underlying left bundle branch block, the catheter may induce complete heart block. In the setting of myocardial infarction, the catheter may induce ventricular fibrillation.
8. Monitor pressures as the catheter is being advanced through the RA, RV, and PA to wedge position. Be careful not to over-wedge.

9. Do not pull back the catheter with the balloon inflated. Damage to valves, either pulmonary or tricuspid may result.

Oximetry Measurements

Oximetry measurements are most commonly performed to measure cardiac output by utilizing the Fick method (described later this chapter) and to rule out a left-to-right shunt (described later this chapter). Oximetry measures the oxygen saturation of blood. The oxygen content of blood can then be calculated.

$$\text{Oxygen Content} \sim \text{Hgb (g/dL)} \times 1.36 \text{ (mLO}_2\text{/g Hgb)} \times \text{Sat}$$

where Hgb is hemoglobin in grams per deciliter, 1.36 is the oxygen-carrying capacity of blood in milliliters of oxygen per gram of hemoglobin, and Sat is the oxygen saturation of the blood. The dissolved oxygen in blood is generally negligible in these calculations and is usually ignored.

Temperature Measurements

A thermistor is mounted at the tip of the pulmonary artery catheter to measure the temperature of the fluid as it passes through the pulmonary artery. Temperature is most commonly used to calculate cardiac output by using the thermodilution technique, which is a variant of indicator dilution. Cold saline is injected through an opening in the catheter 25 to 30 cm proximal to the tip. The temperature is measured as a function of time, and temperature change can be used to calculate cardiac output. (See Cardiac Output section later this chapter.)

Hemodynamic Measurements in Clinical Scenario

Normal hemodynamic parameters (Figures 6-2 through 6-6) and American College of Cardiology/American Heart Association task force recommendations for cardiac catheterization in patients with

FIG. 6-3. Normal right arterial pressures. Right atrial pressure is the same as central venous pressure and is equal to right ventricular diastolic pressure: *a* wave ~ right atrial systole, *x* descent ~ right atrial relaxation, *v* wave ~ right atrial filling during ventricular systole, *y* descent ~ right atrial emptying.

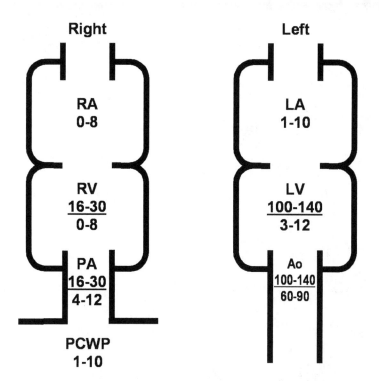

FIG. 6-2. Normal hemodynamic pressure measurements in various cardiac chambers. *RA*, mean right atrial pressure; *RV*, right ventricular pressure; *PA*, pulmonary artery pressure; *PCWP*, pulmonary capillary wedge pressure; *LA*, mean left atrial pressure; *LV*, left ventricular pressure.

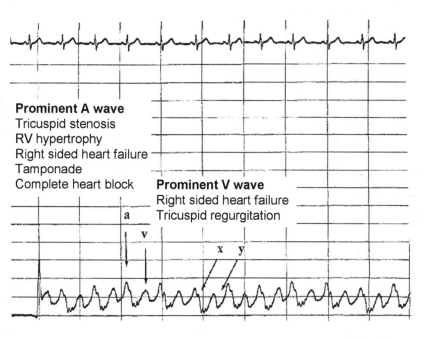

Prominent A wave
Tricuspid stenosis
RV hypertrophy
Right sided heart failure
Tamponade
Complete heart block

Prominent V wave
Right sided heart failure
Tricuspid regurgitation

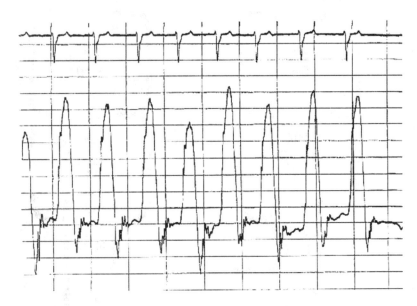

FIG. 6-4. Normal right ventricular pressures. Right ventricular systolic pressures are elevated with right-sided heart failure, pulmonary valve stenosis, and pulmonary hypertension. Right ventricular diastolic pressures are elevated with cardiac tamponade and increased right ventricular stiffness. Note that the distance between horizontal lines is 4 mm Hg and the time between vertical lines is 1 second.

valvular heart disease are listed in Appendixes A and B, respectively.

Pressure Gradients Across Stenoses

Measuring pressure gradients across stenotic valves is an important process in determining the need for surgical intervention, particularly when the hemodynamics, as measured by noninvasive means, are in question. The valve orifice area can often be estimated by a formula that was developed by Dr. Richard Gorlin if the mean pressure gradient, the cardiac output, and the systolic ejection time are known, and if the patient is not in a low cardiac-output state:

$$\text{Valve Orifice Area (VOA) in cm}^2 =$$

$$\frac{\text{Cardiac Output (L/min)}}{44.3 \times (K) \times \text{Heart Rate} \times (\text{SEP or DFP}) \times \sqrt{\Delta P} \text{ (mm Hg)}}$$

where SEP is the systolic ejection period in aortic stenosis (length of time blood is ejected from LV every beat); DFP is the diastolic filling

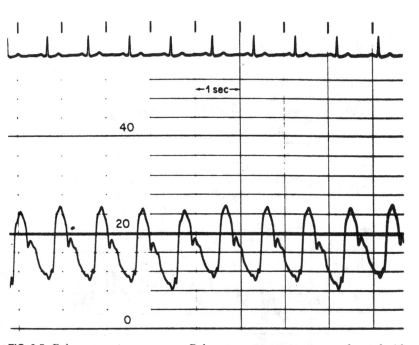

FIG. 6-5. Pulmonary artery pressures. Pulmonary artery pressures are elevated with left sided heart failure, lung disease, and pulmonary vascular disease. In pulmonary vascular disease, the pulmonary artery diastolic pressure can be significantly higher than the pulmonary capillary wedge pressure. This finding is most commonly found in primary pulmonary hypertension, chronic pulmonary embolism, and Eisenmenger syndrome with intracardiac shunts. Note that the distance between horizontal lines is 4 mm Hg, and the time between vertical lines is 1 second. (From Willard JE, Lange RA, Hillis LD. Cardiac catheterization. In: Klonar RA, ed. *The guide to cardiology*, 3rd edition. New York: Wiley Medical, 1995:145–164, with permission.)

period in mitral stenosis (length of time blood fills LV every beat); and DP is the mean pressure gradient. The constant ($K = 0.85$) is factored into the equation in mitral stenosis.

The Hakki formula can be substituted if the heart rate is within normal range:

$$\text{Valve Orifice Area (cm}^2) = \sqrt{\frac{\text{Cardiac Output (L/min)}}{\text{pressure gradient (mm Hg)}}}$$

The Angel correction mandates that the above result be divided by 1.35 for a heart rate of less than 75 beats per minute in the set-

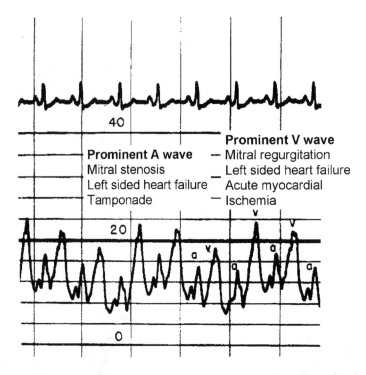

FIG. 6-6. Pulmonary capillary wedge pressures: 'a' wave ~ left atrial systole, 'v' wave ~ left atrial filling during ventricular systole. Note that the distance between horizontal lines is 4 mm Hg, and the time between vertical lines is 1 second. (Adapted from Willard JE, Lange RA, Hillis LD. Cardiac catheterization. In: Klonar RA, ed. *The guide to cardiology*, 3rd edition. New York: Wiley Medical, 1995:145–164.)

ting of mitral stenosis, or greater than 90 beats per minute in the setting of aortic stenosis.

Aortic Stenosis

The normal orifice area of the aortic valve is 3 to 4 cm². The aortic valve can become significantly narrowed prior to the onset of symptoms or even prior to hemodynamic significance.

Aortic Valve Orifice Areas

Normal aortic valve orifice area	3–4 cm²
Mild stenosis	1.1–1.3 cm²
Moderate stenosis	0.8–1.0 cm²
Severe stenosis	<0.8 cm²

The Gorlin formula can be used to estimate the valve orifice area, but may be inaccurate in severe aortic stenosis with low-output states. The accuracy of the formula is flow dependent and will result in small orifice areas, even with low gradients if the flow across the aortic valve is low. To distinguish between "pseudostenosis" and true stenosis, maneuvers to increase the cardiac output can be employed, such as exercise, dobutamine, or nitroprusside. In patients with pseudostenosis, the valve orifice area will increase as flow increases, but it will not change significantly in patients with severe aortic stenosis.

The most accurate method for measuring aortic valve gradients is by obtaining simultaneous pressure measurements from the left ventricle (LV) and the ascending aorta (Figure 6-7). This method allows for the calculation of the mean gradient by direct measurement from both recordings. The two catheters required for this, however, necessitate dual arterial access. A double-lumen pigtail catheter may also be used but is not commonly available. Alternatively, a long arterial sheath can be placed in the descending thoracic aorta, and the pressure measured from the side port. The femoral artery pressure is also often substituted by this

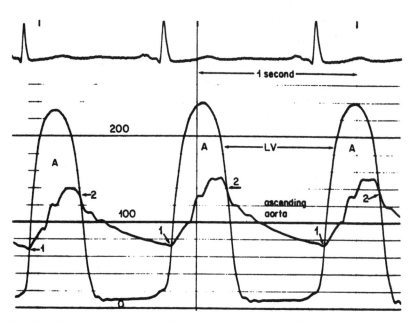

FIG. 6-7. Simultaneous pressure tracings of the left ventricle and the ascending aorta demonstrating a significant gradient across the aortic valve. (From Willard JE, Lange RA, Hillis LD. Cardiac catheterization. In: Klonar RA, ed. *The guide to cardiology*, 3rd edition. New York: Wiley Medical, 1995:145–164, with permission.)

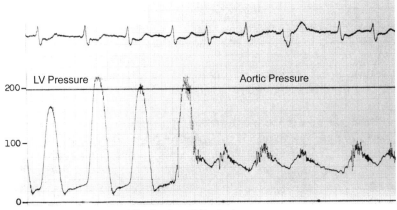

Continuous Withdrawal Tracing from LV to Aorta

FIG. 6-8. Pressure tracing of a pullback across the aortic valve. *LV*, left ventricular.

measurement. The peak femoral artery pressure is usually higher than the peak aortic root pressure due to reflected pressure waves seen in the periphery, thus using the femoral artery results in underestimation of the pressure gradient. This can be somewhat compensated by measuring the pressure difference between the catheter at the ascending aorta and the side arm of the femoral artery sheath, and subtracting the difference.

A more commonly utilized method involves pullback of the catheter from the LV into the ascending aorta. This technique yields a "peak-to-peak" gradient between the maximum aortic pressure and the maximum LV pressure (Figure 6-8). Each of these peaks occurs at different points in time, however, and this measurement is only an estimate of the mean gradient. In addition, in patients with severe aortic stenosis, the catheter itself may take up a significant fraction of the orifice area, resulting in worsened stenosis and increased gradients.

TROUBLESHOOTING

Calculating Valve Area in Aortic Stenosis

68-year-old male:
Cardiac output (CO) = 4,800 mL/min

Heart rate (HR) = 80 beats per minute
Systolic ejection period (SEP) = 0.35
Mean atrioventricular gradient (P) = 80 mm Hg

Gorlin formula:

$$\text{Valve Orifice Area (VOA)} = \frac{CO/(HR)\ (SEP)}{44.3\ (K)\ \sqrt{\Delta P}\ (mm\ Hg)}$$

$$VOA = \frac{4,800/(80)\ (0.35)}{44.3\ (\sqrt{\Delta 80})} = 0.4\ cm^2$$

Hakki formula:

$$VOA = \frac{CO\ (L/min)}{\sqrt{\Delta P}}$$

$$VOA = \frac{4.8}{(\sqrt{\Delta 80})} = 0.5\ cm^2$$

Mitral Stenosis

The normal mitral VOA is 4 to 6 cm². Significant narrowing can occur prior to hemodynamic compromise. When the valve area falls to approximately 2.0 cm², the left atrial pressures will start increasing to maintain cardiac output. Valve areas less than 1.0 cm² may require some intervention.

Mitral Valve Orifice Areas

Normal mitral orifice area	4–6 cm²
Mild stenosis	1.6–2.0 cm²
Moderate	1.1–1.5 cm²
Severe	<1.0 cm²

The gradient across the mitral valve is typically measured with simultaneous measurements of left ventricular (LV) and pulmonary capillary wedge (PCW) pressures as a surrogate for left atrial (LA) pressure (Figure 6-9). The Gorlin equation is also used in this instance, except that the diastolic filling period (Figure 6-10) is used in lieu of the systolic ejection period used in aortic stenosis (AS), and that an empiric constant of 0.85 is added to the equation. Concomitant mitral regurgitation with mitral stenosis will affect this calculation, and usually will underestimate the true orifice area.

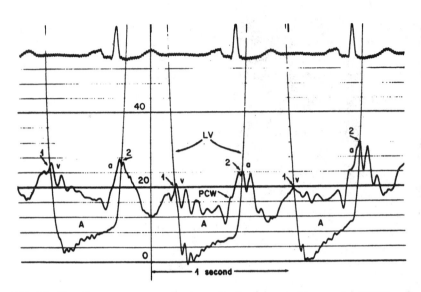

FIG. 6-9. Simultaneous pressure tracings of pulmonary capillary wedge (*PCW*) and the left ventricle pressure demonstrating a gradient across the mitral valve and a slow *y* descent of the PCW pressure tracing. (From Willard JE, Lange RA, Hillis LD. Cardiac catheterization. In: Klonar RA, ed. *The guide to cardiology*, 3rd edition. New York: Wiley Medical, 1995:145–164, with permission.)

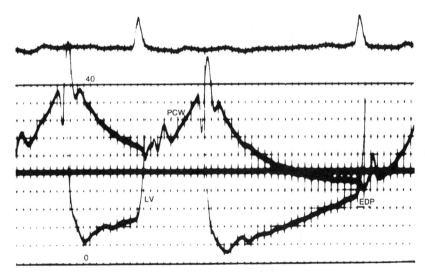

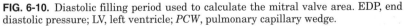

FIG. 6-10. Diastolic filling period used to calculate the mitral valve area. EDP, end diastolic pressure; LV, left ventricle; *PCW*, pulmonary capillary wedge.

TROUBLESHOOTING

Calculating Valve Area in Mitral Stenosis

37-year-old male:
  Cardiac output (CO) = 5,000 mL/min
  Heart rate (HR) = 76 beats per minute
  Diastolic filling pressure (DFP) = 0.4
  Mean mitral valve gradient (P) = 20 mm Hg

Gorlin formula:

$$\text{Valve Orifice Area (VOA)} = \frac{CO/(HR)(DFP)}{44.3 \; (K) \; \sqrt{\Delta P}}$$

where $K = 0.85$ (for the mitral valve)

$$VOA = \frac{5,000/(76)\,(0.4)}{44.3(0.85)(\sqrt{20})} = 1.0 \text{ cm}^2$$

Hakki formula:

$$VOA = \frac{CO \; (L/min)}{\sqrt{\Delta P}}$$

$$VOA = \frac{5.0}{(\sqrt{20})} = 1.1 \text{ cm}^2$$

Hypertrophic Obstructive Cardiomyopathy

In hypertrophic obstructive cardiomyopathy (HOCM), the obstruction lies below the aortic valve and may be dynamic, with little or no resting gradient. The pullback to measure the peak-to-peak pressure should start at the ventricular apex and proceed through the left ventricular outflow tract (LVOT) and through the valve. In typical HOCM, there will be a gradient from the ventricular apex to the LVOT, but no gradient across the valve (Figure 6-11). In Yamaguchi variant, no gradient will be noted, although the classic spade-like appearance may be observed with left ventriculography.

If a significant resting gradient is not appreciated, then provocative maneuvers can be performed to unmask an intraventricular gradient. The most common maneuvers include Valsalva, nitroglycerin administration, isoproterenol administration, amyl nitrite inhala-

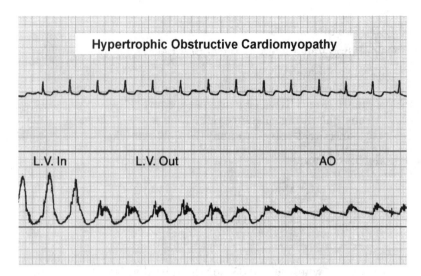

FIG. 6-11. Pullback from left ventricular apex to left ventricular outflow tract demonstrating an intraventricular gradient consistent with hypertrophic obstructive cardiomyopathy. *L.V. In*, left ventricular cavity pressure; *L.V. Out*, left ventricular outflow tract pressure; *AO*, ascending aoritic pressure.

tion, or PVC induction. **The Brockenbrough sign helps differentiate HOCM from valvular aortic stenosis.** In a patient with HOCM, the systemic pressure of the sinus beat following a PVC is lower than that of the sinus beat before the PVC (Figure 6-12).

INTRACARDIAC PRESSURE WAVEFORMS

Mitral Regurgitation

The hemodynamic hallmarks of mitral regurgitation are increased left atrial pressure and reduced cardiac output. A prominant *v* wave is suggestive of, but not specific to, mitril regurgitation (Figure 6-13).

Cardiac Tamponade

A pericardial effusion that results in hemodynamic compromise causes tamponade. With regard to hemodynamic measurements, there is eventual diastolic equalization of pressures (right atrial pressure = right ventricular end-diastolic pressure = left atrial pressure = left ventricular end-diastolic pressure) in all cardiac chambers usually associated with pulsus paradoxus (exaggerated inspiratory fall in arterial pressures of greater than 10 mm Hg), a fall in cardiac output and hypotension. Pulsus paradoxus, however, is neither sensitive nor specific for tamponade, and may be found in constrictive pericarditis, pulmonary embolism, and COPD. On the pressure tracings, there may be a prominent *x* descent with a blunted *y* descent (Figure 6-14).

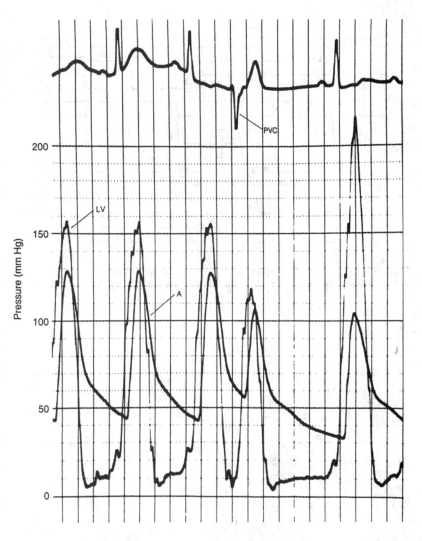

FIG. 6-12. Brockenbrough sign. The gradient across the aortic valve is increased in the post-extrasystolic beat, with a reduction in aortic or systemic pressure. This accentuation of the gradient is either small or absent in a fixed obstruction/valvular aortic stenosis. A, aortic pressure; LV, left ventricle; PVC, premature ventricular contraction.

Constrictive Versus Restrictive Physiology

Making the diagnosis of constrictive pericarditis may be difficult. Differentiating between constrictive pericarditis and restrictive cardiomyopathy is even harder. While the usual features of constrictive pericarditis include elevation and equalization of the diastolic pressures in all four cardiac chambers, a "dip and plateau" pattern in the

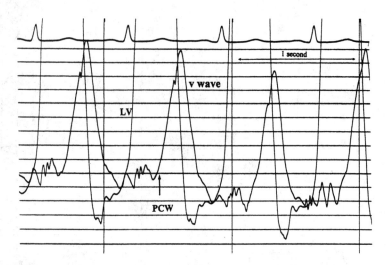

FIG. 6-13. Severe mitral regurgitation. The *v* wave in the pulmonary capillary wedge (*PCW*) pressure tracing is very prominent in this case, and the *y* descent is sharp. *LV*, left ventricle. (From Topol EJ, ed. *Textbook of cardiovascular medicine.* 2nd ed. Philadelphia: Lippincott Williams & Wilkins; 2002, with permission.)

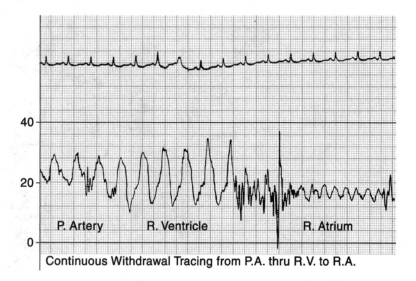

FIG. 6-14. Cardiac tamponade, with a large pericardial effusion. Note the diastolic equalization of pressures in the right ventricular and right atrial positions.

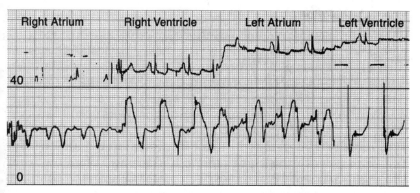

FIG. 6-15. Constrictive pericarditis. A classic "W" or "M" pattern is seen in the right atrial pressure tracing.

ventricular pressure tracings, an "M or W" pattern in the atrial tracing, and an elevation of the mean right atrial pressure during inspiration, none of these features are either sensitive or specific to the diagnosis of constriction. **One finding that may help differentiate between constrictive and restrictive pericarditis is respiratory discordance between the left and right ventricular systolic pressures.** This would require simultaneous pressure recordings in the left and right ventricles (Figures 6-15, 6-16).

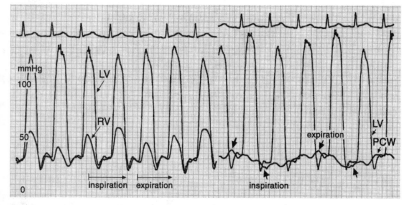

FIG. 6-16. Constrictive pericarditis. Ventricular interdependence and respiratory variation are seen in this example. *LV*, left ventricle; *PCW*, pulmonary capillary wedge; *RV*, right ventricle.

Shunt Calculation

Shunts can be localized and quantified by using oximetry, indocyanine green dye, and angiography. The most common method used clinically is oximetry. In the location of the shunt, blood usually flows from the left-sided (higher-pressure) chamber to the right-sided (lower pressure) chamber (left-to-right shunt), with abnormally high oxygen saturation in that chamber and all chambers distal. The level where this "step-up" is detected identifies where the shunt exists. **A step-up is considered significant if it is greater than 7% from the vena cava to the right atrium and greater than 5% from the right atrium to the right ventricle, or greater than 5% from the right ventricle to the pulmonary artery.**

The quantification of shunting is determined by calculating the shunt fraction, which in left-to-right shunts is the ratio of pulmonary to systemic blood flow (Qp/Qs). Oxygen saturations should be drawn in the superior vena cava (SVC), inferior vena cava (IVC), right atrium (three sites), right ventricle (three sites), pulmonary artery, and aorta.

$$Qp/Qs =$$

$$\frac{O_2 \text{ Sat (systemic arterial)} - O_2 \text{ Sat (systemic mixed venous)}}{O_2 \text{ Sat (pulmonary venous)} - O_2 \text{ Sat (pulmonary arterial)}}$$

Multiplying the SVC saturation by 3, adding it to the IVC saturation, then dividing the sum by 4 calculates the mixed venous saturation.

Minimal Qp/Qs Reliably Detected

1.5–1.9 L/min/m^2 at level of atrium
1.3–1.5 L/min/m^2 at level of ventricle
1.3 L/min/m^2 at level of great vessels

Shunts are small if the Qp/Qs is less than 1.5, moderate if the Qp/Qs is between 1.5 to 2.0 L/min/m^2, and large if the Qp/Qs is greater than 2.0.

TROUBLESHOOTING

Shunt Calculation

61-year-old male with an atrial septal defect and the following oxygen saturations:

Femoral artery = 98% (systemic arterial and pulmonary venous)
Superior vena cava = 69%
Inferior vena cava = 73%
PA = 80%

$$MVO_2 = \frac{(3)\,(0.69) + (0.73)}{4} = 0.70 \text{ (systemic mixed venous)}$$

$$Qp/Qs =$$

$$\frac{O_2 \text{ Sat (systemic arterial)} - O_2 \text{ Sat (systemic mixed venous)}}{O_2 \text{ Sat (pulmonary venous)} - O_2 \text{ Sat (pulmonary arterial)}}$$

$$Qp/Qs = \frac{0.98 - 0.70}{0.98 - 0.80} = 1.55$$

Remember, Qp/Qs:
  <1.5 = small
  1.5–2.0 = medium
  >2.0 = large

Right-to-Left Shunts

Right-to-left shunts cannot be localized or quantified by using a standard right heart catheterization. Sampling must be done at the pulmonary vein level as well as in the chamber of interest (e.g., left atrium) to determine if a "step-down" in saturation is found. This technique usually necessitates a transseptal puncture.

CARDIAC PERFORMANCE

Cardiac Output

The primary purpose of the heart is to deliver oxygenated blood to the peripheral tissues. Cardiac output is measured clinically in two ways: the thermodilution method and the Fick method. Cardiac output can also be indirectly estimated with left ventriculography. Cardiac output is affected by several different factors, including age, body size, and metabolic demands. To normalize resting cardiac output among different body sizes, the cardiac index is used:

$$\text{Cardiac Index (L/min/m}^2) = \frac{\text{Cardiac Output (L/min)}}{\text{Body Surface Area (BSA) (m}^2)}$$

$$\text{where BSA} = \frac{\sqrt{[\text{Height (cm)} \times \text{Weight (kg)}]}}{3,600}$$

Thermodilution Method
The thermodilution technique is based on indicator dilution methods. This method utilizes a bolus injection of a known amount of a substance, and followed by measurement of the concentration of this substance downstream as a function of time. The concentration–time curve can then be used to determine the cardiac output. While this technique has been used with several different indicators, e.g., indocyanine green, **the most common indicator used today is room temperature saline**, with the temperature difference between saline and blood measured in lieu of concentration. The temperature is measured with a thermistor, usually at the level of the injectate bag and at the tip of the catheter. While this usually provides a reasonably accurate result, if the temperature of the saline is increased between the injectate bag and the injection port the measurement can be falsely elevated. This most commonly occurs because the saline is heated by the operator's hand while on the injection syringe. In low-output states, the saline gets warmed by the blood and heart prior to reaching the thermistor, which may result in inaccurate calculations. Valvular abnormalities, such as tricuspid or pulmonic regurgitation, or intracardiac shunting will also affect the thermodilution cardiac output.

TROUBLESHOOTING

Common Pitfalls in Measuring Cardiac Output

1. Warming the saline in the syringe with your hand prior to injection when using the thermodilution method.
2. Not measuring cardiac outputs the same time pressure is measured.

Fick method
In 1870, Adolph Fick developed a principle that demonstrated that **the total uptake or release of any substance by an organ is the product of blood flow to the organ and the arteriovenous concentration difference of the substance.** In common clinical practice, the organ to which this is applied is the lungs, and the substance is oxygen. This method calculates pulmonary blood flow,

which in the absence of intracardiac shunts, equals systemic blood flow. Thus, systemic blood flow equals oxygen consumption divided by the pulmonary arteriovenous oxygen difference. The arteriovenous oxygen difference is calculated by subtracting the oxygen content of mixed venous blood, usually pulmonary arterial blood in most clinical settings, from pulmonary venous blood, which is estimated by systemic arterial blood. The oxygen content equals oxygen saturation (%) multiplied by 1.36 mLO$_2$/g Hgb (oxygen-carrying capacity of hemoglobin) multiplied by hemoglobin (g/100 mL blood). The term for dissolved oxygen in the blood is usually negligible and therefore dropped.

$$\text{Fick Cardiac Output (L/min)} = \frac{\text{Oxygen Consumption (mL/min)}}{(\text{Arterial} - \text{Venous O}_2 \text{ Sat}) \times 1.36 \text{ Hgb (mg/dL)} \times 10}$$

The uptake of oxygen by the lungs can be measured directly by using a metabolic cart. Given the unwieldiness, time, and expense, oxygen consumption is often estimated by a formula or nomogram. This simplification can, however, introduce inaccuracies to the calculation, especially in patients with significantly higher or lower metabolic demands than usual. (See TROUBLESHOOTING: Calculation of Cardiac Output and Cardiac Index.)   •

Factors Affecting Oxygen Consumption

Age
Gender
Hyper or hypothyroidism
Hyper or hypothermia
Exercise
Sepsis

TROUBLESHOOTING
Calculation of Cardiac Output and Cardiac Index

A 56-year-old man:
Height = 180 cm
Weight = 70 kg
Oxygen consumption = 250 mL/min
Arterial oxygen saturation = 98%
Venous oxygen saturation = 70%
Hemoglobin = 14 g/dL

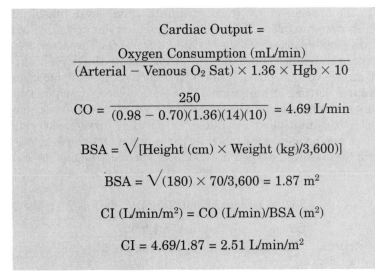

$$\text{Cardiac Output} =$$

$$\frac{\text{Oxygen Consumption (mL/min)}}{(\text{Arterial} - \text{Venous } O_2 \text{ Sat}) \times 1.36 \times \text{Hgb} \times 10}$$

$$\text{CO} = \frac{250}{(0.98 - 0.70)(1.36)(14)(10)} = 4.69 \text{ L/min}$$

$$\text{BSA} = \sqrt{[\text{Height (cm)} \times \text{Weight (kg)}/3{,}600]}$$

$$\text{BSA} = \sqrt{(180) \times 70/3{,}600} = 1.87 \text{ m}^2$$

$$\text{CI (L/min/m}^2) = \text{CO (L/min)}/\text{BSA (m}^2)$$

$$\text{CI} = 4.69/1.87 = 2.51 \text{ L/min/m}^2$$

Angiographic Techniques

This method uses the left ventriculogram to estimate stroke volume based on geometric assumptions about the shape of the ventricle. The stroke volume is multiplied by the heart rate, which gives an estimate of cardiac output. This method usually is the least accurate, especially in ventricles that do not hold up to geometric assumptions (Table 6-2).

Left Ventricular Filling Pressures

The left ventricular filling pressures are often estimated by the PCW pressure. Differentiating between the PA pressure and PCW

TABLE 6-2. **METHODS FOR DETERMINING CARDIAC OUTPUT AND WHEN THEY ARE MOST (OR LEAST) RELIABLE**

Method	Most Reliable for	Least Reliable for
Fick	Low cardiac output	High cardiac output
Thermodilution	High cardiac output	Low cardiac output
		Pulmonic regurgitation
		Tricuspid regurgitation
		Intracardiac shunting
Angiographic	Normal-shaped ventricle	Extensive segmental wall motion abnormalities
		Dilated ventricle
		Aortic regurgitation
		Mitral regurgitation

pressure can sometimes be difficult, especially in the setting of severe mitral regurgitation, but three criteria can be used: **(a) the mean PCW pressure should be about 10 mm Hg less then the mean PA pressure;** (b) blood withdrawn from the catheter in the wedged position should have an arterial saturation; (c) if in the setting of fluoroscopy, the catheter tip is wedged when it is lodged and not moving in the distal PA.

The left ventricular end diastolic pressure (LVEDP) provides the best hemodynamic correlation with the volume status of the heart and can help guide diuretic and vasodilator therapy. The LVEDP in normal patients is 3 to 12 mm Hg. This parameter may increase with pressure or volume overload and with decreased left ventricular compliance.

Potential Etiologies of Left Ventricular End Diastolic
Pressure Elevation

Aortic insufficiency
Mitral regurgitation
Intracardiac Shunts
High-output congestive heart failure
Hypertension
Hypertrophic cardiomyopathy
Aortic stenosis
Cardiomyopathy (ischemic or nonischemic)
Restrictive cardiomyopathy
Infiltrative cardiomyopathy

Vascular Resistance

Resistance is defined as the ratio of the pressure gradient across a vascular bed divided by the flow through that bed. Clinically, the two commonly calculated resistances are the systemic vascular resistance and the pulmonary vascular resistance.

Systemic Vascular Resistance [Wood units (mm Hg/L/min)] =

$$\frac{\text{Mean Aortic Pressure} - \text{Mean Right Arterial Pressure}}{\text{Qs or Cardiac Output}}$$

Pulmonary Vascular Resistance [Wood units (mm Hg/L/min)] =

$$\frac{\text{Mean PA Pressure} - \text{Mean Left Arterial Pressure}}{\text{Qp or CO}}$$

Units: 80 dynes = 1 Wood unit (or mm Hg/L/min)

In most patients, changes in vascular resistance reflect changes in arteriolar tone or changes in the viscosity of blood (often secondary to anemia). In patients who are hypotensive or in shock, systemic vascular resistance (SVR) calculations help to differentiate between certain etiologies, and may help guide therapy. For example, a hypotensive patient with a low SVR may have sepsis, while a patient in cardiogenic shock often has hypotension with an elevated SVR.

SUGGESTED READINGS

Baim DS, Grossman W, eds. *Grossman's cardiac catheterization, angiography, and intervention*, 6th ed. Philadelphia: Williams & Wilkins; 2000.

Bonow RO, Carabello B, deLeon AC, et al. ACC/AHA guidelines for the management of patients with valvular heart disease. *J Am Coll Cardiol* 1998; 32:1486.

Brandfonbrener M, Landowne M, Shock NW. Changes in cardiac output with age. *Circulation* 1955;12:556.

Fick A. Uber die Messung des Blutguantums in den Herzventrikeln. *Sitz der Physik-Med ges Wurtzberg* 1870:16.

Gorlin R, Gorlin SG. Hydraulic formula for calculation of the area of the stenotic mitral valve, other cardiac valves, and central circulatory shunts. *Am Heart J* 1951;41:1.

Hakki AH, Iskandrian AS, Bemis CE, et al. A simplified valve formula for the calculation of stenotic cardiac valve areas. *Circulation* 1981;63: 1050–1055.

Heupler FA. Hemodynamics. Intensive Review of Cardiology Review Course; 2000.

Hurrell DG, Nishimura RA, Higano ST, et al. Value of respiratory changes in left and right ventricular pressures for the diagnosis of constrictive pericarditis. *Circulation* 1996;93:2007–2013.

Kendrick AH, West J, Papouchado M, et al. Direct Fick cardiac output: are assumed values of oxygen consumption acceptable? *Eur Heart J* 1988;9: 337–342.

Selzer A, Sudrann RB. Reliability of the determination of cardiac output in man by means of the Fick principle. *Circ Res* 1958;6:485.

Topol EJ, ed. *Textbook of cardiovascular medicine*, 2nd ed. Philadelphia, PA: Williams & Wilkins; 2002.

APPENDIX A
NORMAL HEMODYNAMIC VALUES

Flows	
Cardiac index	2.6–4.2 (L/min/m$_2$)
Stroke volume index	35–55 (mL/m$_2$)
Pressures (mm Hg)	
Aorta/systemic artery	
Peak systolic/end diastolic	100–140/60–90
Mean	70–105
Left ventricle	
Peak systolic/end diastolic	100–140/3–12
Left atrium (pulmonary capillary wedge)	
Mean	1–10
a wave	3–15
v wave	3–15
Pulmonary artery	
Peak systolic/end diastolic	16–30/0–8
Mean	10–16
Right ventricle	
Peak systolic/end diastolic	16–30/0–8
Right atrium	
Mean	0–8
a wave	2–10
v wave	2–10
Resistances	
Systemic vascular resistance	
Wood units	10–20
Dynes[a]	770–1500
Pulmonary vascular resistance	
Wood units	0.25–1.50
Dynes	20–120
Oxygen consumption	110–150 (mL/min/m$_2$)
AVO$_2$ difference	3.0–4.5 (mL/dL)

[a]The amount of force needed to move a unit weighing 1 g (when acted on continuously) to an acceleration of 1 cm · s^{-2}.
AVO, arteriovenous oxygen difference.

APPENDIX B

ACC/AHA GUIDELINES FOR THE MANAGEMENT OF PATIENTS WITH VALVULAR HEART DISEASE

Indications for Cardiac Catheterization in Aortic Stenosis	Class
1. Coronary angiography before AVRT in patients at risk for CAD	I
2. Assessment of severity of AS in symptomatic patients when AVRT is planned or when noninvasive tests are inconclusive, or there is a discrepancy in clinical findings regarding severity of AS or need for surgery	I
3. Assessment of severity of AS before AVRT when noninvasive tests are adequate and concordant with clinical findings and coronary angiography is not needed	IIb
4. Assessment of LV function and severity of AS in asymptomatic patients when noninvasive tests are adequate	III
Indications for Cardiac Catheterization in Chronic Aortic Regurgitation	Class
1. Coronary angiography before AVRT in patients at risk for CAD	I
2. Assessment of severity of regurgitation when noninvasive tests are inconclusive, or discrepancy in clinical findings regarding severity of regurgitation or need for surgery	I
3. Assessment of LV function when noninvasive tests are inconclusive or discordant with clinical findings regarding LV dysfunction and need for surgery in patients with severe AR	I
4. Assessment of LV function and severity of regurgitation before AVR when noninvasive tests are adequate and concordant with clinical findings and coronary angiography is not needed	IIb
5. Assessment of LV function and severity of regurgitation in asymptomatic patients when noninvasive tests are adequate	III
Indications for Cardiac Catheterization in Mitral Stenosis	Class
1. Percutaneous mitral balloon valvotomy in properly selected patients is performed	I
2. Assessment of severity of MR in patients being considered for percutaneous mitral balloon valvotomy when clinical and echocardiographic data are discordant	IIa
3. Assessment of pulmonary artery, left atrial, and LV diastolic pressures when symptoms and/or estimated pulmonary artery pressure are discordant with the severity of MS by 2D and Doppler echocardiography	IIa
4. Assessment of hemodynamic response of pulmonary artery and left atrial pressures to stress when clinical symptoms and resting hemodynamics are discordant	IIa
5. Assessment of mitral valve hemodynamics when 2-D and Doppler echocardiography data are concordant with clinical findings	III
Indications for Left Ventriculography and Hemodynamic Measurements in Mitral Regurgitation	Class
1. Inconclusive noninvasive tests regarding severity of MR, LV function, or the need for surgery	I
2. Discrepancy between clinical and noninvasive findings regarding severity of MR	I
3. In a patient who has not contemplated valve surgery	III

ACC/AHA, American College of Cardiology/American Heart Association (Task Force on Practice Guidelines); AS, aortic stenosis; AVRT, atrioventricular reciprocating tachycardia; CAD, coronary artery disease; LV, left ventricular; MR, mitral regurgitation; MS, mitral stenosis.

7. HIGH-RISK CORONARY ANGIOGRAPHY

Michael R. Tamberella III and A. Michael Lincoff

The risk of adverse events as a result of coronary angiography is dependent on the underlying coronary anatomy, left ventricular (LV) systolic function, and clinical scenario. The most common reasons for increased risk are listed in Table 7-1.

GENERAL CONSIDERATIONS

Prevention

Certain additional precautions should be taken when the high-risk patient undergoes cardiac catheterization. Ionic contrast agents may cause volume overload, hypotension, bradycardia, anaphylaxis,

TABLE 7-1. CHARACTERISTICS OF HIGH-RISK PATIENTS

Left main coronary artery disease
Severe left ventricular dysfunction
Aortic stenosis
Aortic dissection/aneurysm
Cardiogenic shock
Acute coronary syndrome
Hypertrophic obstructive cardiomyopathy
Severe atherosclerosis of the aorta

contrast nephropathy, and even death. As such, the amount of contrast injected should be minimized.

Two of the most common complications encountered in the catheterization laboratory are hypotension and arrhythmias. **The risk of serious hypotension can be minimized with the judicious use of sedatives, narcotics, and nonionic contrast.** Arrhythmias can be prevented with optimization of electrolytes prior to catheterization. Rapid access to an intraaortic balloon pump (IABP) as well as a temporary pacemaker may prove to be lifesaving.

Early Recognition

Hypotension during catheterization may be secondary to contrast-induced vasodilation, vagal response, ischemia, rhythm disturbances, and hypovolemia. Once hypotension develops, a prompt investigation of potential causes helps guide appropriate management. It is important to ascertain that the apparent blood pressure derangement is not due to artifact, such as catheter damping or catheter whip.

Rhythm disturbances include bradycardia secondary to ionic-contrast or vagal reaction and tachycardia secondary to ischemia, hypotension, electrolyte disturbances, or direct cardiac irritation. Other rhythm disturbances include any degree of heart block, usually secondary to ischemia or direct cardiac irritation.

Management

High-risk patients presenting to the catheterization laboratory are at particular risk for hemodynamic deterioration. Protracted hypotension may require the use of volume expansion with intravenous fluids, vasopressor therapy, and/or IABP placement.

If the cause for hemodynamic collapse is arrhythmia, advanced cardiac life support (ACLS) protocols should be initiated. "Cough cardiopulmonary resuscitation" may help the patient maintain consciousness during a ventricular arrhythmia by accelerating venous return and augmenting cardiac output. However, early defibrillation and initiation of antiarrhythmic medications, such as amiodarone and/or lidocaine, are recommended whenever a patient develops malignant ventricular tachycardia. Continuous infusions of antiarrhythmic medications may be necessary to prevent recurrent arrhythmias.

Transient bradycardia, typically due to ionic contrast agents or hypervagotonia, usually resolves without treatment. Having a patient cough may help clear contrast from the coronary circulation and restore normal heart rate. Significant bradycardia following contrast injections should prompt a switch to nonionic contrast. Bradycardia that does not resolve spontaneously may require treatment with atropine 0.5 to 1 mg i.v. Persistent or recurrent brady-cardia, or high-degree atrioventricular (AV) block unresponsive to atropine, warrants temporary pacemaker placement.

Patients with left bundle branch block (LBBB) are at increased risk of complete heart block during routine right heart catheterization. Contacting the intraventricular septum with the catheter can progress LBBB to complete heart block. Transient first or second-degree heart block is usually managed conservatively. However, if prolonged high-degree AV block occurs in the setting of symptoms, a transvenous pacemaker should be placed.

The risk of myocardial perforation from right heart catheterization increases in patients with thin-walled right ventricles. In patients undergoing right heart catheterization, myocardial perforation is suggested by the paroxysmal onset of ventricular ectopy and hypotension. Fluoroscopic guidance of Swan–Ganz catheters helps prevent right ventricular (RV) free-wall perforation, which may be characterized by an enlarging cardiac silhouette accompanied by shortness of breath, elevated right-sided pressures, and hypotension. **Aggressive volume expansion is usually the only measure needed to support patients with iatrogenic RV perforation.** However, in some instances, echocardiographically guided pericardiocentesis may be necessary.

SPECIFIC DISEASE STATES

Left Main Coronary Artery Disease

According to the Society for Cardiac Angiography and Interventions, patients with left main (LM) coronary artery disease (CAD) have a two-fold greater risk for complications from cardiac catheterization. Angiography of a patient with severe LM stenosis (Figure 7-1) may produce profound hypotension, thereby potentiating myocardial ischemia.

LM disease should be suspected among patients with a markedly positive stress test (LV dilation on stress and/or lung uptake of sestamibi) prior to catheterization, ischemic electrocardiogram (ECG) changes in a large, anterior distribution, or in patients presenting with acute coronary syndromes with associated heart failure. Often, the first clue an operator is provided suggesting LM stenosis is dampening of the catheter upon engagement of the LM ostium (Figure 7-2). If this occurs, the catheter should be promptly removed and carefully reengaged, approaching the LM from a slightly different angle. If dampening recurs and is not rectified with careful catheter manipulation, the catheter should be removed and a subselective injection performed. Injection into the left coronary sinus will often be enough to

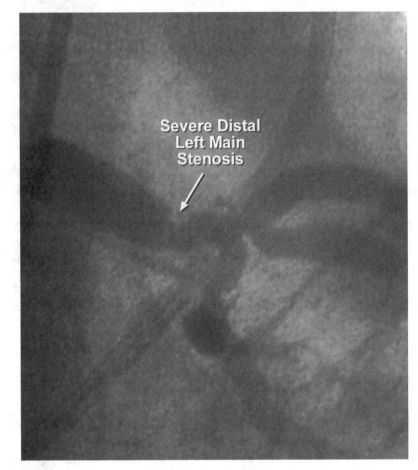

FIG. 7-1. Severe left main trunk (LM) trunk stenosis. Angiogram of the LM trunk at 5-degree right anterior oblique and 36-degree cranial angulation, demonstrating a severe distal LM trunk stenosis (*arrow*).

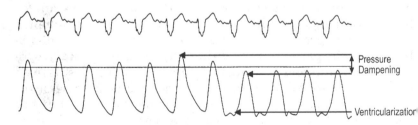

FIG. 7-2. Pressure dampening and ventricularization upon catheter engagement of the left main (LM) trunk. Waveform alterations seen upon catheter engagement of a severe LM trunk stenosis. Clues to LM stenosis include a pressure gradient (damping) and ventricularization of the pressure waveform.

unmask severe disease. **Subsequent injections should be made with nonionic contrast and limited to revealing targets for bypass grafts.** In most cases, the entire study of the left system can be limited to two subselective injections consisting of a straight posteroanterior cranial and a right anterior oblique (RAO) caudal angulated view.

Severe Left Ventricular Dysfunction

Any patient who presents with previously undocumented severe LV dysfunction should undergo left and right heart catheterizations. A thorough test often provides insight towards causality and delineates coronary anatomy. If angiography demonstrates ischemic cardiomyopathy, vessels with the potential to be revascularized can de identified and treated.

Ventricular arrhythmias are especially common in patients with LV dysfunction undergoing heart catheterization. Therefore, rapid access to defibrillators and intravenous antiarrhythmic medications are essential. Following cardioversion, suppressive therapy (usually with amiodarone 1 mg/min infusion or lidocaine 1 to 4 mg/min infusion) should be maintained.

Mild hypotension may be amenable to gentle hydration; however, **care should be taken to avoid volume overload resulting in pulmonary edema.** If hemodynamic instability persists, or if severe CAD is also present, an IABP may need to be inserted. If the patient is volume overloaded upon arrival to the lab, or if congestion develops during the procedure, aggressive use of diuretics and intravenous nitrates is warranted. Echocardiography can supplant left ventriculography to assess cardiac performance and level of valvular disease in these patients.

Severe Right Ventricular Dysfunction

Patients with RV dysfunction and dilation are at increased risk of iatrogenic RV free-wall perforation and should be monitored closely for development of a pericardial effusion. If suspected, emergent echocardiography should be performed to confirm the diagnosis. However, perforations do not routinely require pericardiocentesis unless tamponade or pulseless electrical activity ensues.

Hypertrophic Obstructive Cardiomyopathy

Hypertrophic obstructive cardiomyopathy (HOCM) is a genetic disease with autosomal-dominant inheritance, characterized by hypertrophy of the LV with variable clinical manifestations, and genetic and hemodynamic abnormalities. The main goals of catheterization in patients with HOCM include evaluation of ischemic symptoms despite maximal medical therapy, assessment of left ventricular outflow tract (LVOT) gradient, and delineation of coronary anatomy for patients in whom surgical or percutaneous amelioration of obstruction is contemplated.

Patients with HOCM are at increased risk during cardiac catheterization, predominantly related to the degree of LVOT obstruction. Factors that may increase LVOT obstruction during catheterization relate to a decreased afterload or preload, as well as an increased ventricular contractility. The major complications that may result from increased LVOT obstruction include ischemic chest pain, arrhythmias, hypotension, myocardial infarction (MI), and, rarely, death. When dealing with complications in patients with HOCM, it is important to be cognizant of the fact that potential therapies may seem counterintuitive. For example, the treatment of hypotension in these patients includes the use of beta-blockers. The treatment of congestive heart failure includes the administration of fluids to increase preload and decrease the LVOT obstruction.

These patients comprise a high-risk group of patients in whom incorrect treatment of complications may prove to be lethal.

Aortic Stenosis

The goals of cardiac catheterization in the patient with aortic stenosis (AS) are to confirm the diagnosis of outflow obstruction, localize the obstruction (subvalvular, valvular, or supravalvular), estimate the severity of the stenosis, estimate the LV function, and evaluate the coronary circulation. Patients with AS have an increased presence of aortic root dilation, especially in the setting of a bicuspid aortic valve, which may require alternative catheter selection for selective coronary angiography (see Aortic Dissection/Aneurysm for engaging coronary ostia.) The major complications associated with AS include arrhythmias, myocardial perforation, cardiac tamponade, stroke, MI, and death. **The aortic valve does not need to be crossed if valve surgery is planned on the basis of the noninvasive assessment.** Transient hypotension and/or bradycardia may be lethal in patients with critical AS. In cases of profound and protracted hypotension, IABP counterpulsation may serve as a bridge to definitive therapy. If hypotension occurs while trying to cross the valve, perforation of the coronary sinus with resultant tamponade should be suspected. In such cases, rapid surgical intervention is mandated.

Ventricular arrhythmias are often lethal in patients with severe AS because intravenous medications tend to not circulate well in the setting of severe outflow obstruction. If ventricular fibrillation occurs, ACLS should be initiated and **intracardiac epinephrine** should be given early in the resuscitative effort.

Aortic Dissection/Aneurysm

The goals of cardiac catheterization in patients with a history of CAD and new aortic dissection include assessment of aortic arch and coronary artery anatomy, as well as identification of potential mechanical complications, such as aortic regurgitation, pericardial effusion, and coronary dissection.

It is important to realize that routine angiography in patients without prior revascularization procedures may increase their risk for rupture and tamponade as a result of the time delay. A recent retrospective analysis of 122 patients with aortic dissection and no known history of CAD undergoing surgical repair showed that routine preoperative coronary angiography did not improve survival. On the other hand, those patients with a history of prior surgical revascularization should still routinely undergo preoperative coronary angiography due to increased surgical complexity. **In summary, routine preoperative angiography is recommended for all patients with prior CAD but not necessarily for patients without prior coronary disease.**

Access in a patient with aortic dissection should be carefully thought-out based on all available data. Physical examination that includes documentation of pulses and the presence or absence of pressure differences between arms will assist in planning the optimal approach to catheterization. In addition, knowledge of available imaging studies including computed tomography scans, transesophageal echocardiography, and/or magnetic resonance imaging may improve the safety and success of catheterization in these patients.

A unique catheterization lab complication associated with aortic dissection is extension of the dissection. This typically occurs when the false lumen is inadvertently engaged. Frequent small injections of contrast help identify the location of the catheter. The true lumen usually has brisk pulsatile flow, whereas flow within the false lumen appears static and often fails to clear rapidly. Catheters should be exchanged over a long guide wire to avoid any additional risk for vascular injury.

Engaging the coronary ostia in the setting of ascending aortic aneurysm may be difficult. Use of longer-tipped catheters, like the Judkins (Cook Inc., Bloomington, IN, U.S.A.) left 5 French (F) or 6 catheters (JL5 or JL6) may be necessary to reach the left coronary ostia. Use of the multipurpose catheter may be necessary to reach the right coronary ostia due to effacement of the aortic root.

Acute Coronary Syndromes

The major objective of cardiac catheterization in the setting of an acute coronary syndrome is to identify the culprit lesion(s) and proceed with early reperfusion therapy. These patients are at high risk for life-threatening arrhythmias, cardiogenic shock, and death. In addition, the use of multiple anticoagulant and antiplatelet medications places these patients at higher risk for bleeding and vascular complications. Some operators routinely obtain central venous access prior to arterial access in anticipation of potential complications requiring rapid intravenous therapy. Venous access may also prove helpful if temporary venous pacing becomes necessary (Table 7-2).

Cardiogenic Shock

Patients presenting to the catheterization lab during cardiogenic shock are at very high risk for morbidity and mortality during catheterization. Cardiogenic shock occurs in 5% to 15% of patients with an acute MI. In the GUSTO (Global Utilization of Streptokinase and Tissue Plasminogen Activator for Occluded Coronary Arteries) I trial, patients presenting with cardiogenic shock accounted for 58% of the mortality in the entire trial. The overrid-

---

TABLE 7-2. ACC/AHA INDICATIONS FOR TRANSVENOUS PACEMAKERS IN MYOCARDIAL INFARCTION

Class I
1. Symptomatic bradycardia
2. BBBB
3. New or age-indeterminate bifascicular block with PR-segment prolongation
4. Mobitz type II second-degree AV block

Class IIa
1. New or age-indeterminate RBBB with LAFB or LPFB
2. RBBB with prolonged AV conduction
3. New or age-indeterminate LBBB
4. Incessant ventricular tachycardia for overdrive pacing
5. Recurrent sinus pauses >3 sec unresponsive to atropine

Class IIb
1. Age-indeterminate bifascicular block
2. New or age-indeterminate isolated RBBB

Class III
1. Prolonged AV conduction
2. Mobitz type I second-degree AV block with normal hemodynamics
3. Accelerated idioventricular rhythm
4. BBB or fascicular block known to exist before myocardial infarction

ACC/AHA, American College of Cardiology/American Heart Association (Task Force on Practice Guidelines); AV, atrioventricular; BBBB, bilateral bundle branch block; LAFB, left anterior fascicular block; LBBB, left bundle branch block; LPFB, left posterior fascicular block; RBBB, right bundle branch block.

ing goal of cardiac catheterization in patients with cardiogenic shock is to rapidly identify the coronary lesion(s) responsible.

Most operators will place an IABP prior to angiography to minimize the risk of further hemodynamic collapse. Patients with cardiogenic shock may benefit from routine placement of a pulmonary artery (Swan–Ganz) catheter as well.

Pulmonary Hypertension

Indications for cardiac catheterization in patients with pulmonary hypertension include determination of cause, assessment of severity, localization and quantification of intracardiac shunts, and pulmonary angiography. During any right heart catheterization, the sudden onset of shortness of breath or hypoxemia and hypotension may indicate pneumothorax, pulmonary embolus, or cardiac perforation.

SUPPORT DEVICES

Temporary Pacing

General indications for transvenous pacemaker placement include symptomatic or hemodynamically significant bradycardia secondary to sinus node dysfunction, high-grade AV block, hypervagotonia and significant hypotension associated with AS.

Prophylactic transvenous pacemaker (TVP) placement should also be considered for patients with LBBB who are undergoing right heart catheterization. Aggravating the right bundle may precipitate complete heart block; the overall incidence is about 5% for patients with preexisting LBBB. Patients who develop recurrent and hemodynamically significant atrial arrhythmias during the procedure may benefit from an antitachycardia pacing modality. (Table 7-3).

The most common mode of temporary pacing used in the catheterization lab is transvenous. Transesophageal and transthoracic methods are seldom used. Insertion sites include the femoral, brachial, subclavian, and internal jugular veins, with each site having its own advantages and disadvantages (Table 7-4).

After central venous access has been obtained, the tip of the pacemaker lead is fluoroscopically guided to the right ventricle. The lead is positioned by gentle advancement and torque to the desired fluoroscopic location. The best position for optimizing thresholds and minimizing ectopy is the inferior or septal border of the right ventricle, approximately two-thirds the distance to the apex. The lead should be tested for security by having the patient cough or breathe deeply.

Pacing should be initiated under fluoroscopy. The pacing rate is typically set at ten to 15 beats per minute above intrinsic heart rate.

TABLE 7-3. ADVANTAGES AND DISADVANTAGES OF VARIOUS PACING TECHNIQUES

Pacing Modality	Advantages	Disadvantages
Transvenous	Familiarity by cardiologist Ability to pace multiple cardiac chambers Low capture thresholds Increased duration of pacing	Requires technical skill Invasive technique
Transcutaneous	Ease of applicability Added defibrillation potential	Variable capture Patient discomfort Need for sedation Large pacer artifact
Transesophageal	Relatively noninvasive Involves swallowing pill-sized electrode Paces atrial chambers	Requires specialized equipment Patient discomfort Inability to pace patients with AV node disease
Transthoracic	Quick access	Invasive nature Risk of tamponade, coronary laceration, pneumothorax Poor lead stability

TABLE 7-4. ADVANTAGES AND DISADVANTAGES OF VARIOUS TRANSVENOUS PACER-ACCESS POSITIONS

Access Position	Advantages	Disadvantages
Femoral	Easy access	Leg must be immobilized Patient must lie flat
Brachial	Low-risk local complications Easy to access right ventricle from the left side	Patient must keep arm immobilized or risks dislodgement
Subclavian	Easy access to the right ventricle from the left side Best tolerated by patients after leaving the lab	Risk of pneumothorax Risk of hemothorax if subclavian artery injured Trendelenburg positioning preferred during insertion to avoid air embolus
Internal jugular	Easy access to the right ventricle, especially from the right internal jugular	Risk of pneumothorax and puncture of the carotid artery Trendelenburg positioning preferred during insertion to avoid air embolus

Jerky diaphragmatic movements indicate diaphragmatic pacing, which should prompt pacemaker lead repositioning. The capture threshold, defined as the lowest current necessary for capture, should be established before continuing to the next phase of the procedure. Output is generally started at 5 mA and slowly decreased until capture is lost. If the ventricle is not capture at 5 mA, the lead needs to be repositioned. Once the ideal capture threshold is obtained (<1 mA) the output is set at two to three times the capture threshold. Sensing thresholds are then tested by setting the pacing rate ten to 20 beats below the intrinsic rate, with the pacemaker in its most sensitive setting (lowest millivolt recognition). The sensitivity is then gradually decreased until asynchronous pacing occurs. The pacemaker is then set to sense at 50% of the sensing threshold.

The most common complications of transvenous pacemaker insertion include vascular or myocardial rupture or damage, cardiac tamponade, induction of cardiac arrhythmias, pneumothorax, and bleeding complications at the access site.

Intraaortic Balloon Pump (IABP)

Indications and contraindications of IABP placement are listed in Table 7-5. When first introduced in 1962, IABPs were surgically placed. Beginning in 1980, however, the percutaneous approach via the femoral artery replaced the surgical approach as the primary means of insertion. **Balloon size is selected based on the patient's height. Most patients receive a 40-cc balloon. Patients shorter than 64 in. or taller than 72 in. require smaller (34 cc) or larger (50 cc) balloons, respectively.** The IABP can be inserted either through a sheath (8F or 9.5F catheter) or via a sheathless technique.

After vascular access has been obtained, the IABP is inserted into the descending thoracic aorta over a guide wire. Fluoroscopic guid-

TABLE 7-5. INDICATIONS AND CONTRAINDICATIONS FOR INTRAAORTIC BALLOON PUMP PLACEMENT

Indications	Contraindications
Cardiogenic shock	Moderate aortic insufficiency (>2+)
Severe mitral regurgitation	Abdominal aortic aneurysm
Decompensated aortic stenosis	Aortic dissection
Ventricular septal defect	Bilateral lower-extremity PVD
Refractory ischemia	Significant arteriovenous shunts
High-risk PCI	Severe coagulopathy
Bridge to definitive therapy	Sepsis
	No planned, definitive therapy

PCI, percutaneous coronary intervention; PVD, peripheral vascular disease.

ance is essential to achieving optimal placement in the aorta. The proximal radiopaque tip should be located just below the subclavian artery or at the level of the carina (Figure 7-3), and the distal end should be above the renal arteries (usually at the level of L1-2) and completely out of the sheath. The central lumen is aspirated and flushed with heparinized saline and connected to a pressure transducer. The balloon is then connected to the pump and filled to one-half the volume. Adequate filling and location should be confirmed by fluoroscopy. Once location is confirmed, the IABP is filled completely and then secured with sutures. Patients are routinely placed on systemic

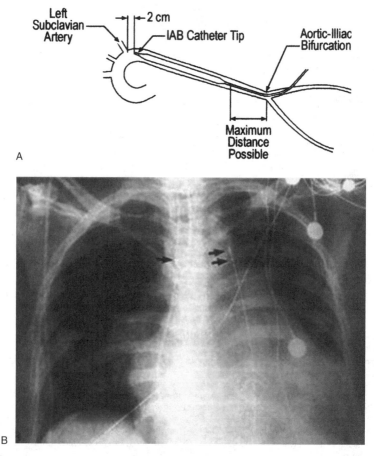

FIG. 7-3. Optimal positioning of the IABP. **A:** Diagram demonstrating the optimal positioning of the intraaortic balloon pump (*IAB*) pump (IABP) approximately 2 cm distal to the left subclavian artery. **B:** The radiopaque tip of the IABP is located approximately 2 cm cranial to the left mainstem bronchus at the level of the carina (*double arrowheads*).

anticoagulation to prevent potential thromboembolic complications resulting from an indwelling intravascular device. However, manufacturers of IABPs insist systemic anticoagulation is optional.

Optimal adjustment of the timing and triggers results in maximum hemodynamic effects (Figure 7-4). Timing of inflation should

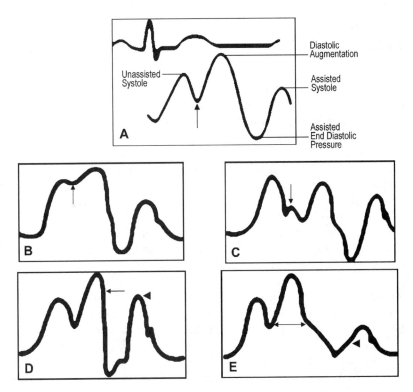

FIG. 7-4. Timing of intraaortic balloon pump (IABP) inflation and deflation. **A:** Correct timing. With correct timing of IABP inflation and deflation an augmentation of diastolic and systolic blood pressures is seen. Inflation occurs at the onset of diastole (*arrow*) and deflation should occur prior to the onset of systole (*arrowhead*) resulting in decreased aortic end-diastolic and systolic pressures. **B:** Premature inflation. Inflation of IABP prior to dicrotic notch (*arrow*). This may result in premature aortic valve closure, increased left ventricular (LV) wall stress, aortic regurgitation and increased myocardial oxygen demand. **C:** Delayed inflation. Inflation of IABP following the dicrotic notch (*arrow*) may result in inadequate accentuation of coronary perfusion. **D:** Premature deflation. Observed as a precipitous drop in the pressure waveform following diastolic augmentation (*arrow*). Other observations include a suboptimal diastolic augmentation and an assisted systole that is equal or greater than the unassisted systole (*arrowhead*). This may result in suboptimal afterload reduction and increased myocardial oxygen demand. **E:** Delayed deflation. Observed as an assisted end diastolic pressure equal to or greater than the unassisted end diastolic pressure, a prolonged rate of rise of the assisted systole (*arrowhead*) and a widened diastolic augmentation (*double arrow*). A lack of afterload reduction and an increase in myocardial oxygen demand occurs.

TABLE 7-6. COMMON COMPLICATIONS ASSOCIATED WITH INTRAAORTIC BALLOON PUMP COUNTERPULSATION

Vascular ([a]6%–25%)	Nonvascular ([a]4%–15%)
Hematoma formation	Sepsis
Arterial dissection	Thrombocytopenia
Vascular laceration	Hemolysis
Limb ischemia	Groin infection
Thromboembolic complications	Peripheral neuropathy
Renal ischemia	
Spinal cord ischemia	

[a]Incidence.

correlate with the onset of diastole. To properly adjust timing of inflation, the IABP should be placed on an inflation ratio of 1:2 to observe augmented and unaugmented beats. The central pressure waveform is used to guide proper timing. Ideally, the balloon should inflate with the closure of the aortic valve, identified by the dicrotic notch of the central pressure waveform tracing. Deflation should occur with aortic valve opening, which can be timed with the onset of the R wave by ECG tracing. When timed appropriately, the central aortic waveform should have an augmentation pressure greater than the systolic pressure, and a postdeflation pressure 10 to 15 mm Hg below the unaugmented diastolic blood pressure.

After IABP insertion, patients should have daily checks of hemoglobin, hematocrit, platelet count, white blood cell count, renal function, and a chest x-ray for placement. Meticulous attention to peripheral pulses and access site are of paramount importance in detecting early vascular complications.

Complications can be divided into vascular and nonvascular. (Table 7-6) Vascular complications occur in 6% to 25% of cases. Specific complications include limb ischemia, arterial dissection, vascular laceration (requiring surgical repair) and major hemorrhage.

SUGGESTED READINGS

Bertrand ME. Identification of intervention patients at increased risk. *Am Heart J* 1995;130:647–650.

Boehrer JD, Lange RA, Willard JE, et al. Markedly increased periprocedure mortality of cardiac catheterization in patients with severe narrowing of the LM coronary artery. *Am J Cardiol* 1992;70:1388–1390.

Penn MS, Smedira N, Lytle B, et al. Does coronary angiography before emergency aortic surgery affect in-hospital mortality? *J Am Coll Cardiol* 2000;35:889–894.

8. HEMOSTATIC DEVICES

B. Keith Ellis and A. Michael Lincoff

Devices
  Manual or Mechanical Compression
  Biosealant
  Collagen Plug
  Vascular Sandwich
  Percutaneous Suture
Advancements

Femoral artery closure devices are being used more frequently in an effort to improve patient comfort, lower costs, and decrease complications associated with femoral artery cannulation for cardiac catheterization. These devices offer the advantages of early sheath removal and hospital discharge, as well as allow for uninterrupted anticoagulation, if needed. The currently available vascular closure devices fall into one of five categories: 1) manual or mechanical compression, 2) biosealant, 3) collagen plug, 4) vascular sandwich involving a collagen sponge and polymer anchor, and 5) percutaneous suture, with minimal variation in cost between devices (from $175 to $190 at our institution).

Important vascular complications associated with femoral arterial puncture and their associated clinical and procedure-related risk factors are listed in Table 8-1 and Table 8-2, respectively. The risk of vascular complications requiring surgery ranges from 0.5% to 1% following diagnostic catheterization, from 1% to 3% following balloon angioplasty, and up to 11% following coronary stenting. **Although randomized trials of closure devices have not demonstrated a significant reduction in vascular complications for any single device,** they improve patient comfort and shorten hospital length of stay.

TABLE 8-1. **POTENTIAL VASCULAR COMPLICATIONS**

Pseudoaneurysm
Arteriovenous fistula
Hemorrhage
Thrombosis
Embolism
Infection

TABLE 8-2. RISK FACTORS ASSOCIATED WITH INCREASED INCIDENCE OF VASCULAR COMPLICATIONS

Clinical Risk Factors
    Advanced age
    Female sex
    Smaller body-surface area
    Congestive heart failure
    Peripheral vascular disease

Procedural Risk Factors
    Anticoagulation
    Cardiac intervention (percutaneous transluminal coronary angioplasty, atherectomy, valvuloplasty)
    Use of larger-sized sheaths

DEVICES

Manual or Mechanical Compression

Manual or mechanical compression remains the gold standard for obtaining hemostasis following femoral artery puncture and is still regularly used whenever femoral artery dissection or hematoma occurs, or per patient request. For patients who have just undergone percutaneous intervention, or in those who have been on anticoagulation with heparin, manual compression can be safely performed once the activated clotting time (ACT) is less than 180 seconds or the activated partial thromboplastin time is less than 50 seconds.

Manual pressure is held directly over the femoral artery at a point proximal to the sheath entry site. **Pressure should be held for approximately 3 minutes per French catheter** size for arterial punctures and 2 minutes per French catheter size for venous punctures, and can be gradually reduced over that time. Patients typically remain supine from 4 to 8 hours after hemostasis is achieved, although some data suggest patients may safely ambulate as early as 2.5 hours after manual compression. Large series of patients undergoing cardiac catheterization have noted major vascular complication rates of ≈0.23% with manual compression. Limitations include the length of time required before ambulation, prolonged hospitalization time, patient discomfort, the need to interrupt anticoagulation therapy while maintaining hemostasis, and the need for trained personnel.

The SyvekPatch (Marine Polymer Technologies, Danvers, MA, U.S.A.) is made of poly-N-acetyl glucosamine, which causes local vasoconstriction and potentiates clot formation. This small patch should be applied directly over the arterial puncture site and manually compressed for 10 minutes following sheath extraction. ACT should be less than 300 seconds. Patients are required to lie supine for 2 hours after the patch has been held in place. The SyvekPatch does not require the insertion of any foreign material into the body, and it allows for immediate repeat arterial puncture if necessary. Other advantages include shortened hospitalization, and a low incidence of major vascular complications (0.1%).

Mechanical compression involves the use of a C-arm clamp, sandbags, or a pneumatic compression device (Femstop, RADI Medical Systems, Uppsala, Sweden). The C-arm clamp is a device with a flat base and a horizontal arm that extends over the base, and angles down at 90 degrees to apply pressure to the femoral artery. The tip of the device consists of a metal or plastic disc, which is placed directly over the arterial puncture site for approximately 20 to 30 minutes. The Femstop applies direct pneumatic pressure over the femoral artery to tamponade bleeding. A transparent plastic bubble is placed over the arterial puncture site, and secured with a plastic arch and belt wrapped around the patient (Figure 8-1).

A recent study that compared manual to mechanical compression demonstrated that time to hemostasis was approximately 33% shorter with manual compression. **Patients are required to lie in the supine position for a period of 4 to 8 hours following**

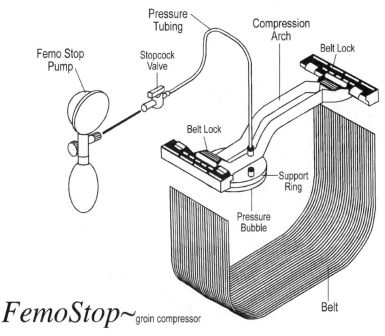

FIG. 8-1. Graphic depiction of the Femstop device for vascular hemostasis. This type of mechanical compression device places a transparent plastic bubble over the arterial puncture site and secures it with a plastic arch and belt wrapped around the patient. (Courtesy of RADI Medical Systems, Inc., Reading, MA, U.S.A.)

either manual or mechanical compression. Studies done in the 1970s and 1980s have shown that there were no significant differences in rates of vascular complications between manual and mechanical compression techniques. Although mechanical compression devices provide a hands-free approach, they do not eliminate the need for staff supervision during the period of compression.

Biosealant

Biosealant devices (Duett, Vascular Solutions, Inc., Minneapolis, MN, U.S.A.) should only be used when arterial access was obtained with a single, anterior puncture of the common femoral artery. This device incorporates a balloon-positioning catheter in combination with a biologic procoagulant mixture of collagen and thrombin (Figure 8-2). The

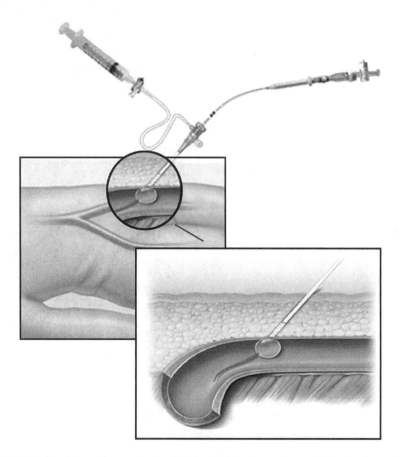

FIG. 8-2. The Duett closure device. Balloon-positioning catheter within the femoral artery and attached syringe of procoagulant mixture. Balloon tamponade of arteriotomy while procoagulant is injected into tissue surrounding puncture site (inset).

balloon-catheter-sealing device is advanced through the femoral sheath, inflated, and then retracted into the puncture site. The procoagulant mixture of collagen and thrombin is injected to the tissue surrounding the arterial puncture site. The sheath is removed, the balloon is deflated, and manual pressure is applied for 2 minutes. **Patients are required to remain in the supine position for approximately 2 hours** to promote adequate hemostasis and reduce the risk of complications. **A delay of 90 days before repeat arterial puncture is not required with the use of the Duett device.** A large study comparing the Duett device to manual pressure showed that the times to hemostasis and ambulation were significantly lower with the Duett device, but that the incidence of major vascular complications was higher.

Collagen Plug

Collagen plugs (VasoSeal, Datascope Corporation, Mahwah, NJ, U.S.A.) can be used interchangeably with biosealant devices. To deploy this device, a dilator and sheath are collectively advanced over a guide wire to the surface of the femoral artery (Figure 8-3), the dilator is removed, and collagen is injected through the sheath into the vascular access track. **Following placement of the device, patients are kept supine for 2 hours.** In patients undergoing coronary angiography, the VasoSeal device had mean times to hemostasis and ambulation of 18 minutes and 110 minutes, respectively. However, some studies (Sanborn et al., 1993) have noted an **increase in vascular complications following** percutaneous coronary intervention.

Vascular Sandwich

A vascular sandwich (AngioSeal, St. Jude Medical, Inc., Minnetonka, MN, U.S.A.) involves placing a collagen plug directly over an intravascular anchoring system. Initially, a carrier sheath is exchanged for the femoral artery sheath (Figure 8-4). Once inserted, the intravascular anchor protrudes from the end of the carrier into the femoral artery. The sheath and carrier are then removed, which pulls the intravascular anchor against the inside of the arterial wall. Tension is applied to the connecting suture, advancing the collagen plug down onto the outside of the arterial wall defect. **The patient is required to remain in the supine position for 2 hours after the AngioSeal has been deployed. Repeat arterial puncture should not be performed for a period of 90 days.** With regards to safety and efficacy, a randomized trial comparing the AngioSeal to manual pressure showed that time to hemostasis following angiography was significantly shorter in the AngioSeal

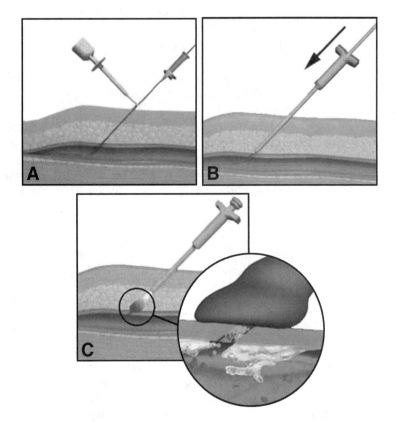

FIG. 8-3. The VasoSeal closure device. **A:** Measurement of depth to arteriotomy. **B:** Dilator advanced over guidewire to previously demarcated depth at surface of femoral artery. **C:** Collagen injected over arteriotomy site while simultaneously withdrawing delivery apparatus resulting in vascular hemostasis **(inset)**.

group (2.5 minutes) compared with the manual pressure group (15.3 minutes). This study also demonstrated significantly fewer complications, such as bleeding and/or hematoma formation, for AngioSeal patients receiving heparin. In general, the AngioSeal device affords rapid deployment, earlier hospital discharge, and improved patient comfort following cardiac catheterization. It also has the lowest reported vascular complication rates of all closure devices.

Percutaneous Suture

Percutaneous suture devices include Prostar, Techstar, and Perclose (Abbott Laboratories, Redwood City, CA, U.S.A.) (Figure 8-5). **These devices are advantageous for patients with large arterial punctures, procedures requiring uninterrupted**

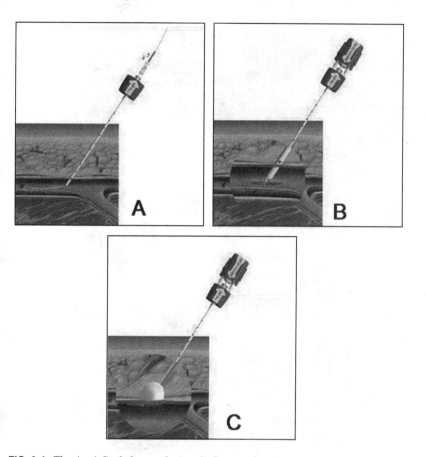

FIG. 8-4. The AngioSeal closure device. **A:** Carrier sheath inserted over a guidewire into vascular lumen. Blood flow through vessel locator verifies correct intra-vascular positioning. **B:** Device inserted into artery with anchor exposed. Note arrow-to-arrow design of this device ensures correct insertion. **C:** Collagen plug and anchor "sandwich" the arteriotomy site with the use of the tamper tube.

anticoagulation, or for whenever repeat arterial access is anticipated. The device deploys needles from inside the arterial puncture site, which are delivered through the subcutaneous tissue and tied. A knot pusher is then used to advance the knot to the arterial wall. **Following the placement of the percutaneous suture, patients are required to remain in the supine position for 1 to 2 hours.** A trial comparing four different methods of arterial closure showed that the Perclose had a 2.3% incidence of major complications, inferior only to AngioSeal. Another large randomized trial found that the times to hemostasis, ambulation, and

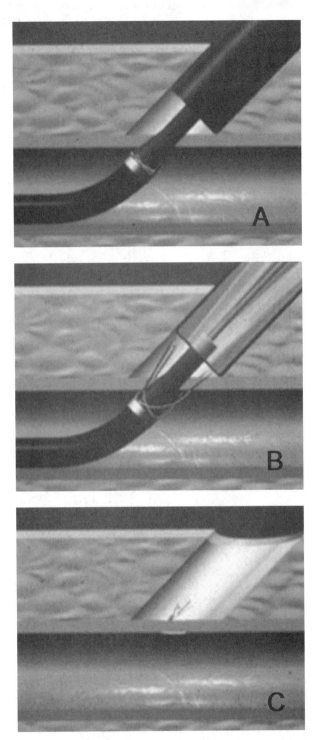

FIG. 8-5. The Perclose closure device. **A:** Perclose system within femoral artery. **B:** Deployment of suture. **C:** Hemostasis achieved with tamping of knot down to arteriotomy

discharge were significantly lower in patients who received suture-mediated closure compared to manual pressure. The mean time to ambulation was 2 hours with suture-mediated closure, and 6.5 hours with manual compression. However, a significantly higher incidence of vascular complications was noted in the suture-mediated closure group. Anticoagulated patients derived particular benefit from suture-mediated closure in regards to hemostasis, time to ambulation and discharge.

ADVANCEMENTS

The 6 French (F) catheter system via the femoral artery remains the most widely used system for coronary angiography. However, operators are increasingly using 4F and 5F catheter systems to shorten hospitalization time. In fact, larger sheath size has been shown to directly correlate with the incidence of groin complications. A recent study involving coronary angiography patients noted that the **mean time from sheath removal to ambulation was approximately 2 hours using a 4F catheter system**. The major limitation of smaller sheath size is suboptimal coronary angiography.

CONCLUSION

Vascular closure devices enhance patient comfort after angiography and/or interventions, and improve overall cath lab efficiency. However, these advantages come with a price. Specifically, the use of vascular closure devices is associated with a greater risk of hematoma, hematocrit drop (greater than 15%), and vascular surgery.

SUGGESTED READINGS

Baim DS, Knopf WD, Hinohara T. Suture mediated closure of the femoral access site after cardiac catheterization: results of the suture to ambulate and discharge (STAND I and STAND II) Trials. *Am J Cardiol* 2000;85: 864–869.

Bogart A. Time to hemostasis: a comparison of manual versus mechanical compression of the femoral artery. *Am J Crit Care* 1995;4:149–156.

Carey D, Martin JR, Moore CA. Complications of femoral artery closure devices. *Cathet Cardiovac Intervent* 2001;52:3–7.

Chamberlin JR, Lardi AB, McKeever LS. Use of vascular sealing devices (Vasoseal and Perclose) versus manual compression (Femstop) in transcatheter coronary interventions requiring Abciximab (Reopro). *Cathet Cardiovac Intervent* 1999;47:143–147.

Dangas G, Mehran R, Kokolis S. Vascular complications after percutaneous coronary interventions following hemostasis with manual compression versus arteriotomy closure devices. *J Am Coll Cardiol* 2001;38:638–641.

Ellis SG, Moone M, Talley, JD. Duett femoral artery closure device vs manual compression after diagnostic or interventional catheterization: results of the SEAL Trial. *Circulation* 1999;100:I-513.

Kussmaul III WG, Buchbinder M, Whitlow PL. Rapid hemostasis and decreased access site complications after cardiac catheterization and angioplasty: results of a randomized trial of a novel hemostatic device. *J Am Coll Cardiol* 1995;25:1685–1692.

Nader RG, Garcia JC, Drushal K, et al. Clinical evaluation of the SyvekPatch in consecutive patients undergoing interventional, EPS and diagnostic cardiac catheterization procedures. *J Invas Cardiol* 2002;14: 305–307.

Sanborn TA, Gibbs HH, Brinker JA, et al. A multicenter randomized trial comparing percutaneous collagen hemostasis device with conventional manual compression after diagnostic angiography and angioplasty. *J Am Coll Cardiol* 1993;22:1273–1279.

Shrake KL. Comparison of major complication rates associated with four methods of arterial closure. *Am J Cardiol* 2000;85:1024–1025.

Sola R, Pastore GM, Stein B. Early ambulation after diagnostic cardiac catheterization: A 4 French study. *J Invas Cardiol* 2001;13:75–78.

Wood RA, Lewis BK, Harber DR, et al. Early ambulation following 6 French diagnostic left heart catheterization: a prospective randomized trial. *Cathet Cardiovasc Diagn* 1997;42:8–10.

9. POST-CATH

Hitinder S. Gurm and A. Michael Lincoff

Local Complications
    Hematoma
    Retroperitoneal Hematoma
    Pseudoaneurysm
    Arteriovenous Fistula
    Infections
Physical Limitations Following Catheterization
Indications for Routine Labs

Although a relatively safe procedure, cardiac catheterization carries a low but significant risk of both major and minor complications. A postcatheterization evaluation should focus on detecting signs and symptoms of possible complications following the procedure.

A brief history should be elicited to detect any symptoms suggestive of catheterization complications (Table 9-1). The postcatheterization examination accordingly needs to focus on the most likely complications and should be directed by the history. The vital signs should be reviewed and blood pressure and pulse checked in supine and erect position.

The jugular venous pressure should be assessed as an index of intravascular status, while cardiac auscultation should focus on the presence of a pericardial rub. All patients who have had subclavian or jugular cannulation need to be examined for signs of pneumothorax, as it may not manifest during the procedure.

The presence of tachycardia after cardiac catheterization should always prompt a search for the underlying cause. It may be due to a manifestation of intravascular depletion, decompensated heart failure, or pericardial irritation. Fever immediately after catheterization is not likely to be related to the catheterization, but it may be a pyrogen reaction to fluids or medications. A new fever should, however, always prompt a search for an infective focus.

A brief neurologic examination is typically performed before discharge. Special attention should be paid to the patient's speech and gait. Importantly, patients may not note neurologic deficits until they ambulate; these may include focal paresis or paralysis, visual symptoms, sensory deficits and ataxia.

TABLE 9-1. SYMPTOMS SUGGESTIVE OF CARDIAC CATHETERIZATION COMPLICATIONS

Symptom	Differential Diagnoses
Chest pain	Coronary ischemia
	Aortic dissection
	Coronary perforation
	Cardiac perforation
Dyspnea	Coronary ischemia
	Congestive heart failure
	Pneumothorax
Groin pain	Localized bleeding
Leg pain/numbness	Femoral nerve compression
	Femoral artery dissection
	Femoral artery thrombosis
	Local nerve block from anesthetic
Flank pain	Retroperitoneal bleed
Nausea/hiccups	Hemopericardium
Blurred vision, unilateral weakness, dysphasia	Cerebrovascular accident

LOCAL COMPLICATIONS

The most important part of the post-cath check is the examination of the catheterization site. **Patients should be examined for evidence of bleeding, pseudoaneurysm, arteriovenous fistula (AVF), or vascular compromise.** Distal pulses need to be carefully assessed, and the femoral artery should be palpated and auscultated for bruits. Due to their associated morbidity, three local complications — bleeding, pseudoaneurysm, and infection — will be discussed in greater detail.

Hematoma

Bleeding after cardiac catheterization may manifest as a hematoma. Clinically, hematomas present as pain or focal discomfort, discoloration, and bruising, and rarely present as femoral nerve compression with resultant quadriceps weakness.

Factors associated with an increased risk of local bleeding include advanced age, female sex, low body mass index (BMI) and use of anticoagulants or platelet glycoprotein IIb/IIIa inhibitors Carefully monitoring anticoagulation therapy helps reduce this risk Hemostasis should be achieved with manual pressure or a mechanical compression device (i.e., Femstop, RADI Medical Systems Uppsala, Sweden) before leaving the patient's bedside.

Retroperitoneal Hematoma

A retroperitoneal hematoma is usually associated with arterial puncture above the inguinal ligament. Multiple punctures, and puncture through the posterior wall of the artery, will dramatically increase the risk of bleeding. Since all the bleeding may be internal, the patient often presents with unexplained hypotension and tachycardia. While flank pain and bruising may be seen in some patients, an unexplained fall in hematocrit may be the only finding in others.

The best modality for detection of a retroperitoneal hematoma is a computed tomography (CT) scan. Ultrasound may be used if CT is not available. Since the therapy of retroperitoneal hematoma is based on its clinical implications and directed towards correcting them, some physicians do not routinely obtain radiologic imaging studies. Instead, they reserve these for patients in whom a definitive diagnosis is required to guide therapy, such as determining the need for withholding anticoagulant or antiplatelet therapy.

TROUBLESHOOTING
Management of Retroperitoneal Hematoma

The mainstay of therapy for a hematoma or retroperitoneal hematoma consists of volume resuscitation and blood transfusion if needed. Anticoagulants and platelet antagonists should be withheld. The decision to reverse anticoagulation and transfuse platelets in patients receiving platelet glycoprotein IIb/IIIa inhibitors or platelet ADP antagonists (ticlopidine or clopidogrel) has to be individualized for each patient.

Pseudoaneurysm

A pseudoaneurysm is defined as an arterial wall disruption with resultant extra luminal flow into a chamber contained by adjacent tissue. Arterial endothelium does not comprise the interior of the pseudoaneurysm. **The incidence of pseudoaneurysm is between 0.3% to 0.5% of cardiac catheterizations.** In a recent study of patients treated with platelet glycoprotein IIb/ IIIa inhibitors, pseudoaneurysms were noted in 0.5% of patients treated with manual pressure, 0.8% of patients treated with AngioSeal, and 0.4% of patients treated with Perclose.

A pseudoaneurysm may manifest as pain, a bruit, a pulsatile mass, an expanding hematoma, and/or leg weakness. The majority arise from the common femoral artery. The best diagnostic imaging modality for a pseudoaneurysm is color flow Duplex ultrasonography. Rarely, they may rupture or lead to thromboembolism, neurovascular compression, or pressure necrosis. **Risk factors include multiple arterial punctures, superficial femoral artery puncture, larger sheath size, hypertension, and the use of antithrombotic therapy.**

TROUBLESHOOTING

Management of Femoral Artery Pseudoaneurysm

Ultrascan guided thrombin injection (UGTI) is the preferred method of treatment in most cases. A recent large series reported a success rate of 94%. Ultrasound guided compression was the most commonly used therapy prior to the advent of UGTI, but it was associated with a relatively high failure rate of 5% to 15%. Similarly, surgical repair has been associated with a high risk of complications. There have been small case series of successful use of endovascular-covered stents to treat pseudoaneurysms.

Arteriovenous Fistula

AVFs occur in approximately 0.11% to 0.16% of diagnostic catheter-izations and in 0.87% of percutaneous coronary interventions, irrespective of hemostatic technique. AVFs develop when the needle tract crosses both the femoral artery and vein and is then dilated during sheath insertion. Risk factors include an arterial puncture below the common femoral artery, larger arterial sheath size, older age, and prolonged anticoagulation or fibrinolytic therapy.

An AVF is clinically characterized by a continuous bruit at the site of catheter insertion. In addition, an expanding groin hematoma, decreased or absent lower-extremity pulses, and a pulsatile mass in the groin may be appreciated. Diagnosis of an AVF is confirmed by Doppler ultrasound.

TROUBLESHOOTING

Management of Arteriovenous Fistula

Small or asymptomatic AVFs can often be monitored with serial ultrasound evaluations. Indications for intervention include a lack of spontaneous closure, increased fistula size, or development of symptoms. Although interest in percutaneous techniques for closure of AVFs is increasing, surgical repair remains the gold standard as fistulae tend to enlarge over time.

Infections

Groin infection is a rare complication of cardiac catheterization. This is rarely seen with manual compression (reported incidence, 0.05%), but its incidence is higher in patients receiving closure devices (0.3%). The most commonly implicated organism is *Staphylococcus aureus*. Patients may present with groin pain, erythema, purulent discharge, fever, and leucocytosis. The proposed access site should be carefully inspected prior to insertion of a sheath, and an alternate site should be selected if there are concerns about dermal integrity. While some physicians administer periprocedural prophylactic antibiotics to patients receiving closure devices, no randomized controlled data supports such therapy. The lack of proven benefit must be weighed against the risk of drug allergy, superinfection, drug resistance, and cost.

The therapy for groin infection consists of appropriate antibiotics and surgical debridement, if indicated. Early consultation with a vascular surgeon is advisable.

PHYSICAL LIMITATIONS FOLLOWING CATHETERIZATION

All patients are advised to restrict activities for a short duration of time to permit adequate healing of the access site. Table 9-2 outlines commonly prescribed minimum restrictions for patients after cardiac catheterization. Some patients may be advised to restrict their activities further based on the findings of their cardiac catheterization.

INDICATIONS FOR ROUTINE LABS

No labs need to be checked routinely after diagnostic cardiac catheterization. In patients suspected of bleeding, the hematocrit

TABLE 9-2. ACTIVITY RESTRICTION FOLLOWING CARDIAC CATHETERIZATION

Approach	Activity Restriction
Brachial	Dressing can be removed after 1 day
	No strenuous activity for 48 h or until sutures removed (cut down):
	No lifting of objects >10 lb
	No activity involving excessive pushing or pulling with affected arm (i.e, no bowling or tennis)
Femoral	No swimming or bathing (can shower) for a week if closure device used
	For the first 24 h:
	No driving
	No lifting of objects >10 lb
	No climbing, cycling, or similar activity involving the lower extremities

should be checked as necessary. Renal function can be checked after 48 hours in patients with renal insufficiency, especially if they are taking metformin or are otherwise suspected to be at higher risk for contrast-induced nephropathy.

SUGGESTED READINGS

Aguirre FV, Topol EJ, Ferguson JJ, et al. Bleeding complications with the chimeric antibody to platelet glycoprotein IIb/IIIa integrin in patients undergoing percutaneous coronary intervention. EPIC Investigators. *Circulation* 1995;91:2882–2890.

Applegate RJ, Little WC, Craven T, et al. Vascular closure devices in patients treated with anticoagulation and IIb/IIIa receptor inhibitors during percutaneous revascularization. *J Am Coll Cardiol* 2002;40: 78–83.

Cherr GS, Travis JA, Ligush J Jr., et al. Infection is an unusual but serious complication of a femoral artery catheterization site closure device. *Ann Vasc Surg* 2001;15:567–570.

Cooper CL, Miller A. Infectious complications related to the use of the angio-seal hemostatic puncture closure device. *Catheter Cardiovasc Interv* 1999;48:301–303.

La Perna L, Olin JW, Goines D, et al. Ultrasound-guided thrombin injection for the treatment of postcatheterization pseudoaneurysms. *Circulation* 2000;102:2391–2395.

Lumsden AB, Miller JM, Kosinski AS, et al. A prospective evaluation of surgically treated groin complications following percutaneous cardiac procedures. *Am Surg* 1994;60:132–137.

Thalhammer C, Kirchherr AS, Uhlich F, et al. Postcatheterization pseudoaneurysms and arteriovenous fistulas: repair with percutaneous implantation of endovascular covered stents. *Radiology* 2000;214:127–131.

Waigand J, Uhlich F, Gross CM, et al. Percutaneous treatment of pseudoaneurysms and arteriovenous fistulas after invasive vascular procedures. *Catheter Cardiovasc Interv* 1999;47:157–164.

SUBJECT INDEX

Page numbers followed by *f* indicate figures; those followed by *t* indicate tables.

A

Abdominal aorta, anatomy of, 65*f*

ACC (American College of Cardiology), guidelines for management of patients with valvular heart disease of, 110

Access needle, 27–28

Acetylcysteine (Mucomyst), for renal dysfunction, 13, 14*t*, 24

Activity restriction, post-cath, 139, 139*t*

Acute coronary syndrome. *See* Acute myocardial infarction

Acute marginal branches, 39

Acute myocardial infarction cardiac catheterization for, 3–6, 4*t*, 5*t*, 118
indications for transvenous pacemakers in, 118, 118*t*

Additives, to contrast agent, 20*t*

AHA (American Heart Association), guidelines for management of patients with valvular heart disease of, 110

Air, elimination from system of, 41

Air embolism
due to coronary angiography, 53
due to left ventriculography, 78*t*

ALARA (as low as reasonably achievable) principle, 25, 26*t*

AL (left Amplatz) catheter, 30–32, 31*f*

Allen test, 35, 36

Allergic reaction(s)
during cardiac catheterization, 12–13
to contrast agents, 2, 13, 23*t*, 24
to latex, 2

to medications, 2
to procaine, 35

American College of Cardiology (ACC), guidelines for management of patients with valvular heart disease of, 110

American Heart Association (AHA), guidelines for management of patients with valvular heart disease of, 110

Amiodarone, after cardioversion, 115

Amplatz catheters
for coronary angiography, 30–32, 31*f*, 42, 43
for left ventriculography, 71

Anaphylactoid reactions, to contrast agents, 23*t*, 24

Anemia, as contraindication to cardiac catheterization, 9–11

Aneurysm
aortic
coronary angiography with, 117
history of, 1
post-cath pseudo-, 137–138

Angina
Canadian Cardiovascular Society classification of, 6, 6*t*
as indication for cardiac catheterization, 4*t*, 5*t*, 6, 9*t*
unstable
as indication for cardiac catheterization, 9*t*
risk factors with, 7–8, 7*t*

Angiographic catheter. *See* Catheter(s)

AngioSeal closure device, 130–131, 130*f*